SWEET SECRETS

Stories of Menstruation

Each time I have a period — and that has only been three times — I have the feeling that in spite of all the pain, unpleasantness, and nastiness, I have a sweet secret, and that is why, although it is nothing but a nuisance to me in a way, I always long for the time that I shall feel that secret within me again.

— Anne Frank,
The Diary of Anne Frank

SWEET SECRETS

Stories of Menstruation

by

KATHLEEN O'GRADY
AND PAULA WANSBROUGH

CANADIAN CATALOGUING IN PUBLICATION DATA

Main entry under title:
Sweet secrets: stories of menstruation

Includes bibliographical references and index.
ISBN: 0-929005-33-3

1. Menstruation – Juvenile literature. 2. Menstruation – Juvenile fiction. I.
O'Grady, Kathleen, 1967– . II. Wansbrough, Paula, 1965 – .

QP263.S83 1997   j612.6'62   C97-931634-0

"Blood" is reprinted from Jane Eaton Hamilton's
collection of short fiction, *July Nights*.

"Outrunning Gravity" by Mary Helen Stefaniak first appeared in
Redbook magazine in August 1985 under the title "Little Girl Lost."

"Blood and Chestnuts" by Kathleen O'Grady first appeared in
Voices and Echoes: Stories and Poems of Women's Spirituality, Jo-Anne Elder
and Colin O'Connell (editors) (Wilfrid Laurier University Press, 1997).

Edited by Rhea Tregebov
Copyright © 1997 by Kathleen O'Grady and Paula Wansbrough

*Second Story Press gratefully acknowledges the support of the Ontario Arts Council
and the Canada Council for the Arts for our publishing program.*

Cover illustration by Laurie Lafrance
Printed and bound in Canada

Published by
SECOND STORY PRESS
*720 Bathurst Street Suite 301
Toronto, Ontario
M5S 2R4*

To every girl
who has ever been
confused, excited, scared, annoyed and *proud*
about having her period.

CONTENTS

Reaching Out

The Challenge

The Passage

Putting It All Together

Acknowledgements

Many individuals and organizations have participated in the development of this book and deserve our gratitude. Generous grants from the Canada Council for the Arts and the Ontario Arts Council made much of our research possible. As well, we would like to thank the Wilfrid Laurier University Women's Centre, the Wilfrid Laurier Graduate Students' Association and the Wilfrid Laurier University Graduate Studies and Research Department for providing early financial backing for initial stages of this project. And for helping us complete this book, we thank the wonderful women of Second Story Press, especially Rhea Tregebov and Karen Farquhar.

Throughout the entire project the inhabitants of the Department of Religion and Culture at Wilfrid Laurier University have championed our efforts. In particular, great thanks goes to Cathie Huggins, departmental office administrator, for her limitless enthusiasm and assistance. Professors Harold Remus, Peter Erb, Ron Grimes, Stephanie Walker, Kay Koppedrayer, Bob Fisher and Michel Desjardins provided continuous editorial, ethnographic and publicity advice, and were unceasingly confident in our ability to create and publish this book. In the project's conceptual stages, Sandra Woolfrey of Wilfrid Laurier Press offered advice on publishing procedures, while roving reporter Jim Boyce instigated media interest. Thanks also to Jessica Harrod of St Stephen's Community House, Toronto, for encouraging young women to participate in the collection and to Betty Cushing and the senior women of Conestoga Lodge, for their wise words and participation.

Dedication and enthusiasm from a number of remarkable people accentuated the pleasures of this project. Janice Shaw, Marie Kelly, Susan Deiter, Christine O'Grady and Mark Logan assisted with proofreading and publicity, and offered valued commentary and analysis. Others have helped by continuously bolstering our spirits, in particular Carolyn Saunders, Viveka von Rosen, Rubina Ramji, Cindy O'Grady, Ken Paradis, Kristine Wendell, Mary Johnston, Myrna Logan, Doreen Broadbent, Rob Wansbrough, Jennifer Dumpert, Stephan Dobson and Kerry Winter. Paul Kelly surrendered his Macintosh LC while the manuscript was developed and supplied Paula with lots of support during moments of angst and exhaustion. Mark Logan endured Kathy's sometimes obsessive behaviour and erratic enthusiasm with great love, wisdom and patience. We are especially appreciative of our parents, Marg and Sandy Wansbrough, and Marlene and Ron O'Grady, for passing on to us their open, frank and positive understanding of health and sexuality, and their respect for the strength and knowledge of women.

There were many invaluable books that helped us along the way. Of special importance were The Boston Women's Collective's *Our Bodies, Our Selves,* Thomas Buckley and Alma Gottlieb's *Blood Magic,* Emily Martin's *The Woman in the Body,* and Judy Blume's *Are You There, God? It's Me, Margaret,* which infused our work with strength and vivacity.

And finally, we applaud all of those people who wrote or submitted work to the collection. Without the courage and creativity of each of these individuals, this book would never have materialized.

— *Kathleen O'Grady & Paula Wansbrough*
August 1997

Dear Reader,

Welcome to Sweet Secrets!

Facts are important; they can explain how and why things like periods happen. But facts aren't able to explain everything. Sometimes we need other ways to help us understand life, especially when things start to change and the world gets a little confusing. So along with all of the facts, this book also contains short stories by women who describe what happened to them, how they felt and what they did around the time of their first periods.

We think that you will learn just as much from these stories as you will from the facts. And if you read them together, you can't miss!

But let's face it. This is a big book and there is no way you're going to sit down and read through the whole thing from cover to cover in one sitting. Well, don't worry! We don't expect you to.

We suggest that you go straight to what interests you most. You may want the facts right away. If so, flip to THE INSIDE STORY where you'll find all the details about what's going on inside your body. Or maybe you prefer to read about the experiences of others. In that case, you'll probably want to skip to the stories and read them first. You could read every word from the first page to the last; or you may decide to read the whole thing backwards!

We've provided a few tools to help guide you through this book. There's a CONTENTS page at the beginning which lists all of the different sections in the book; it may help you to decide what to read first, but then again, you may just want to flip through on your own.

There's also a handy GLOSSARY near the end of this book. If you're looking for a specific word that you don't understand, maybe a word like "cervix," or if you want a basic description of something, let's say "ovulation," then this is the place to look. And if you're interested in a particular topic, for instance, "tampons," then just flip to the back of the book, and the INDEX will tell you what pages cover this topic.

You'll also find a section at the end that describes the different women who've helped make this book. ABOUT THE AUTHORS contains interesting information about the women who wrote the stories. We also interviewed many women, from ages thirteen to ninety-three, and included their thoughts about menstruation in MENSTRUATION FACTS. You can find out more about these women in the ABOUT THE OTHER CONTRIBUTORS section.

At the back of the book, you'll find a CALENDAR. Use the calendar to keep track of the days that you menstruate. It's a kind of mini, period diary. Over the months, this will give you a picture of your menstrual cycle. Soon you'll see if your body has any regular patterns.

All together, we hope that this book will help make your first period a wonderful moment, full of excitement and pride. And we hope that every time you menstruate, you'll learn something new about the mysteries of your body.

Welcome to the world of women! Good luck, and happy reading.

From Paula and Kathy

MENSTRUATION

FACTS

☉

Beginnings

@

What's It All About?

THIS BOOK IS ALL ABOUT the bleeding that we women do from the special opening between our legs. As you may already know, such bleeding is called "menstruation," "having your period," "your time" and lots of other names.

There's something magical about menstruation. There are explanations why menstruation occurs, but no one seems to fully understand all of the different and mysterious aspects of women's bleeding.

Did you know that women who live in the same house or who see each other often, like close friends or relatives, often start to menstruate on exactly the same day, in "synchronicity"? Or that for thousands and thousands of years women have used the phases of the moon as a way to mark the passage of their bleeding cycles? And that many cultures all over the world treat menstruation as a powerful and sacred process? First menstruation is an especially important event and has been celebrated by people throughout history.

But what will having a period mean for *you*?

First menstruation signals that your body is *slowly* getting ready for sexual activity and having babies. But there's more to it than just that. The beginning of menstruation, and of growing breasts and pubic hair, also means that you're becoming an adult, transforming like a caterpillar into a butterfly!

Already you're growing taller and you're probably wanting more respect from the people around you. You're sick of being treated like a child and feel ready to take on the world, wear what you want and be with your friends. Menstruation is a special part of this complicated package of growing up, gaining independence and becoming your own person.

Your First Period

It's difficult to know for certain when your first period will arrive. Some girls are as young as eight or nine when they begin menstruating. Other girls don't get their periods until they're sixteen or seventeen. Our individual bodies are all unique and mature in slightly different ways and at different speeds. You may feel like you've been waiting forever when you finally discover that first spot of blood in your underwear. Or you may not think that you're ready, but your body will be!

> When I first started bleeding I had no idea what was going on. I thought I was really sick because my mom had never told me about it. Even she didn't expect me to get it that early. I was so tiny — my maxi-pad was three times bigger than I was.
>
> *Rubina Ramji (age 29)*

> Mom told us we'd be late menstruating because that's the way it was in our family. She hadn't menstruated until seventeen years — and I was sixteen.

I so wanted to be like the other girls. They had breasts and I remember one who was most popular. The boys flocked around her. She wore sweaters all the time and had beautiful round breasts.

I'll never forget the first time. We had a basketball game. We won and when I changed I had that wonderful brown stain on my panties. I wasn't embarrassed. I padded myself well with toilet paper and hurried home. I burst in on Mom, told her — she smiled and said, "I guess you're ready for the glad rags, dear."

Ruth Helliwell (60s)

Find out from your mom or your sisters or your parents' sisters (they're all *blood* relations) when their first periods arrived. Because you're biologically related, there may be a similarity in the way you'll mature.

If you're adopted or if you're looking for other clues, you can estimate when your first period will arrive by paying close attention to your body's growth. Usually your first period will come after you've grown armpit hair and pubic hair (that curly stuff between your legs), after your hips and breasts have developed some, and after you've grown taller rather suddenly. You may also notice that your hair and skin are oilier and that your underarm odour is stronger. All of these things are signs that you're experiencing PUBERTY — those years of rapid growth and change that will transform you from a kid into an adult.

However, sometimes periods are the earliest signs of puberty and come as a surprise. You can prepare yourself for the Big Day by carrying a pad in your schoolbag and by learning what you can about your body's changes.

"I Want It But I Don't!"

Just as we start our periods at different ages, we also have different feelings about menstruation. Some girls can't wait to have that first period and check daily to see if they've started menstruating yet. They're excited by the thought of growing up. Other girls pretend it will never happen to them and avoid talking about menstruation. And when we get our periods, some of us feel strong and healthy and proud about being women. Others find menstruating messy and embarrassing, or just a big pain.

I think my menstrual blood is beautiful. At first it's dark red, then bright red, then pink, then brown and then it fades away. I also like the way it feels when it's leaving my body.

My period is part of me. I've been menstruating for sixteen years already and I'll be menstruating for many years to come. It's because of these years that we spend having periods that we need to go back to celebrating this significant change in our lives. When my daughter begins menstruating she is going to have a celebration, even if it's only between her and me.

Roberta Kennedy (30s)

When you're a child, you struggle to have a clean and perfect body and then, with menstruation, everything springs out of control. There is mess. There are leakages. There are strange new smells. You don't know when it is going to happen. There is pain, deep, achy pain in the very centre of your body. With the thick pad wagging between my legs, I felt that I had gone back to diapers. I was sure everyone would know and I was ashamed. Was this what it meant to be a woman? I experienced my first period as a loss of power, not as a gain, a return to babyhood, not an entry into adulthood.

Elizabeth Mossman (30s)

You may be excited and want to get your period on the one hand, but on the other hand think that it's a disgusting and weird thing. Having contradictory feelings about menstruating is normal.

People Can Be Weird and Wonderful

When you begin to menstruate you may find that some of your family relationships change. This is because you may feel and act differently, or because people see you in a new way, or both!

Some parents are just wonderful when their daughter first begins to menstruate. They're proud and happy, calm and helpful. Your parents may show their appreciation of your new maturity by giving you added responsibilities and freedoms. They may take some special time to explain the changes in your body to you, or, if they're shy or don't feel they know all of the answers, they might give you books and other information to help prepare you.

Parents may also act very awkwardly when their daughter has her first period. They may feel that their "little girl" is growing up. They're scared she won't need them any more and frightened about all of the adult things that she's going to want to do. And they might not know what words to use to explain their mixed feelings. You may see some strange responses from the people around you, even from the people you love the most. It's hard for many adults to change, so be patient!

When I first got my period, Mom bought me a jumbo-sized box of pads, a stretchy elastic belt for the pads and a jar of green olives with pimento centres. I love olives and this jar was all mine. When my sister got her period, we were all relieved because it seemed late in coming. Mom treated my sister and me to a celebration dinner. We slurped up spaghetti in a rich tomato sauce and we toasted her period with red wine, clinking our glasses, whispering, giddy, giggly. We finished the meal with cheesecake topped with glistening red strawberries.

Athena George (30s)

I got my first period during Hockey Night in Canada. After Mother and I sorted things out, I returned to the hockey game, stomach cramping, nursing my new knowledge on the couch. Later, during third period, after Dad had gone upstairs for a swig of Coke, he came back and said, "Mom says you've got your period. That's great!" and he smiled.

Diane Driedger (30s)

Before I got my first period, I began to notice strange events. My sister — who is eighteen months older than I — was hiding things from me. She and my mother would go to the pharmacy together and secretively bring things home. There would be something in a bag, although I don't think I ever saw a pad. My sister would go to the washroom and would be hiding something when she came out. When I asked, she said, "You'll find out some day."

When I began menstruating, my mother began to talk constantly about the interactions between girls and boys. I was not to be friendly with boys, go out with them or even go to school dances.

Esmeralda Carvalho (20s)

Roll Out the Red Carpet!

Periods confuse a lot of people. Men and women you know who are normally smart or easy to talk to and up-front about even the most difficult topics may become ashamed and embarrassed by menstruation. They just don't know what to say or how to say it even though they know it's important stuff. They act this way because there are a lot of wrong ideas that menstruation is dirty and bad. Menstruation is *not* bad and it is *not* dirty. It is not an illness or a disability either, but a normal and important part of a woman's life cycle that shows her every month that her body's healthy.

I often think that it is ignorant that we don't speak out more about menstruation. Those are things that should be talked over with the children. Mothers or sisters should tell one another. Other girls never mentioned it to me. And I had no sisters, you see. And I certainly wouldn't go to my brothers and ask them because I knew I was different than them. Years ago everything was hushed up. I was frightened when I started menstruating. I thought I was haemorrhaging. Everything was hushed up, as though it was something dirty. It's not dirty. It's natural!

Ursula Kroft (90s)

I really regret that many of us are not taught that our periods are cleansing. Our blood flows through our bodies every month to clean out our uterus and our vagina. What a concept! We are not experiencing "the curse" as I was taught when I first started my menses. We are not "dirtying" our pads and tampons. And when we do have accidents, we're not "dirtying" our underwear or our sheets.

I also regret that our periods are not, as yet, a cause for celebration. When a young girl begins her menses a big celebration would be fine! I feel these celebrations should be international holidays. For one special day every year, women all over the world would be honoured because of our periods. Maybe we could have parades of women marching the streets with floats of red. Red streamers, red flowers. Maybe that's too much. But I think this holiday would need to be recognized by a parade, or rally, or a woman's dance. Or perhaps a party of red with a lot of singing and dancing.

Roberta Kennedy (30s)

❂ Beginnings ❂

Unfortunately many people have not been taught that menstruation is a natural and good thing and they fear it because they don't understand the process. Sometimes this fear causes people to make jokes and rude remarks about menstruating women — most of which are not even based on the facts! Be prepared for some silly, even mean responses from people, and if you can, try to teach them the truth about menstruation.

It's a Woman's World!

Around the time of your first period, you may discover how important your friends and sisters are to you. Some of the best people to talk to about menstruation are girls your own age. You can share tips with your friends, like which pads or tampons are best, or find out how to cure menstrual cramps from your favourite cousin. Sometimes you'll discover that you and your friends have your periods at exactly the same time! You can learn from your friends and you can teach them the things that you've discovered too.

On the other hand, most boys know very little about menstruation — for some strange reason many adults don't think it's necessary to explain this stuff to them. Boys often feel uncomfortable about periods. Some boys will make nasty jokes while others will be embarrassed when girls talk openly about bleeding.

Jeananne: If you want to make guys uncomfortable, you just start talking about menstruation.

Janti: If you want them to go away you start talking about your period and they run!

Maja:	But it's weird how it varies in guys. Kurt went *looking* for "fem-i-nine hy-giene pro-ducts" in my bag!
Susan:	That was the day you had about eight hundred in the front pocket of your bag.
Maja:	And today we were in the variety store and he was going through my bag and he said, "Eww! Used ones!" I'm like, "*What* are you talking about! We don't keep them after!"
Susan:	Didn't Joel one time think you only got it once or something?
Maja:	Once a year. He thought you got it only once a year!
Janti:	Once a year! We're like, "Please, please, please!"
Maja:	But then you'd probably get it for, like, *two months.*
Jeananne:	Imagine having it for *two months.*

Susan, Janti, Jeananne and Maja (ages 13 – 14)

Boys' odd reactions come from a fear of what they do not know. You can have fun with it, like Jeananne, Janti, Maja and Susan. Or keep bleeding a secret between the girls. If you're feeling very patient, you might even want to teach a boy a fact or two!

What's in a Name?

There are lots of different names for your bleeding time. Doctors like to use scientific names and so they call it "menstruation" or "menses," terms that come from the Latin word *mensis* which means "month." Some moms and grandmas think it's polite to say "that time of the month," "your monthlies," or "your time." There are also mystical names that celebrate your natural cycle: "moontime" is the most common, but some people also call their bleeding "moonflowers" or "redrose."

There are angry names too, like "the curse," for those days when you aren't happy about menstruating. People who don't appreciate the importance of menstruation have called it a curse as if it's a bad spell or something horrible. Certainly there are times when menstruation seems to get in the way, but more often it's a blessing, a sign of good health, maturity and womanliness.

Another name, "on the rag" ("OTR"), describes what women used in the past to catch their blood. Before cotton pads could be bought in stores, women wore cloth rags that they washed and reused every month. Today some people still say that they are "on the rag."

Both names — "on the rag" and "the curse" — are sometimes used as put-downs when a woman is moody, angry or assertive by people who have the confused idea that menstruation makes women go crazy. These people think women should always be sweet, quiet and meek. When a woman doesn't act the way they think she should, they believe something is wrong with her and place the blame on the very thing that makes her most womanly — the fact that she can bleed and have babies.

There are also many names for menstruation that can be fun and friendly: "Aunt Flo," "Aunt from Red Bay," "the little man" and "my friend" are all "visitors" that come to call every month.

And finally there's the most common term — "period." This name can fit almost any mood. It refers to a cycle that repeats over and over again like class periods in school, or it can mean the end of a cycle, just like the period at the end of this sentence means that the sentence is finished.

If you're not happy with any of these names for your bleeding time, be creative and come up with one of your own! Share this new name with your friends or keep it as a special secret.

THE INSIDE STORY

◎

First, What's on the Outside?

FIRST MENSTRUATION IS A great time to learn about your body, inside and out.

As you know, women and men have different GENITALS — the "private parts" between their legs. Genitals are often called SEX ORGANS or REPRODUCTIVE ORGANS because they're the parts of our bodies that we use when we have sex and when we have babies. Men's sex organs hang outside their bodies: the PENIS and the sac called TESTICLES. Women's sex organs are both inside and outside and are much more complicated.

Women's genitals — the outside sex organs — are also called the VULVA. This is the area between your legs; it will change a lot as you go through puberty. The folds and lips of skin called LABIA will become softer and looser. You'll grow curly PUBIC HAIR. And every month or so, menstrual blood will drip out of the special opening between your labia. This opening is the entrance to the VAGINA. We'll talk more about the vagina later.

Besides the vaginal opening, there are two other openings or holes protected by the folds of your labia and by your buttocks. The first is the URETHRA. It's from here that you urinate (pee). The other opening is the ANUS. It's from this hole that you have bowel movements (poo, do number two).

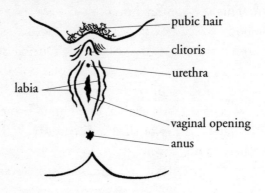

pubic hair

clitoris

urethra

labia

vaginal opening

anus

The Main Characters

The inside story of menstruation has many characters, like the characters in a play. Each organ or part of your body has a different role to play and must learn to work in harmony with the rest.

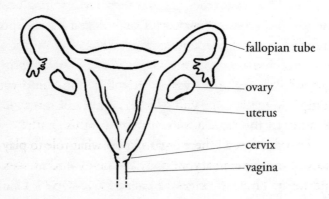

fallopian tube

ovary

uterus

cervix

vagina

◉ The Inside Story ◉

An important player in the menstruation story is the VAGINA. This is a spongy tunnel that leads from the outside of your body to the sex organs inside. Menstrual blood and babies come out through the vagina. During sexual intercourse, a man's penis is slid into a woman's vagina. You can look at the opening of your vagina if you hold a mirror between your legs. Your vaginal opening is protected by the labia and may be damp or slick to the touch.

Another main character maturing in your body right now is your UTERUS or WOMB. It's a very strong, muscular organ. The uterus is about the size of your fist and is hollow. When a woman is pregnant, the uterus holds the developing baby and expands like a balloon as the baby grows. Hold your closed fist against your lower stomach right below your belly button to see where your uterus is located.

To the left and right of your uterus are thumbnail-sized organs called OVARIES. Ovaries are powerful places. They hold hundreds of thousands of tiny EGGS, also known as OVA. Even before you were born, you had these eggs in your ovaries.

The CERVIX is the gate between your vagina and your uterus. You can see your cervix only if you have a speculum (an instrument that opens up your vagina) and mirror to look into, but you can feel your cervix if you carefully push your finger far up into your vagina. It will be the bump your fingertip will meet at the end of your vagina and it may be quite sensitive to your touch, so be sure to try this gently!

In order that all these organs know what role to play in the story of menstruation, your body and brain send messages back and forth. These messages are called HORMONES. Like actors reading the script for a play, your sex organs read hormones to know what to do next. Hormones are always flowing through your body, but there are many more of them during puberty when your body is maturing and learning new processes and sensations. The hormones ESTROGEN and PROGESTERONE are the messages for the process of menstruation. These two hormones are called the female sex hormones.

The Amazing Menstrual Cycle: A Step-By-Step Process

A cycle is a process that repeats itself over and over again. Your first period signals that an amazing cycle has begun. The menstrual cycle is made up of different stages all directed by those busy hormones. Usually when we think of our menstrual cycle, we think only of the time when we're bleeding. But just because you can't see things happening doesn't mean your reproductive organs are just sitting around doing nothing!

During the first stage of the menstrual cycle, your uterus grows a blood lining inside itself. The fancy name for this lining is ENDOMETRIUM. The endometrium grows and thickens for a week or so until the next event, OVULATION, takes place.

Ovulation is the point in your cycle when an egg is squirted out from your ovary. Your ovaries take turns releasing eggs — usually only one ovary lets out one egg per cycle. During the next three to five days, the egg travels down one of the passages called the FALLOPIAN TUBES on its way from your ovary to your uterus. Some women say that they can tell when they're ovulating because they feel particular things, like a twinge to the right or left of their bellies, rushes of creativity, or strong emotions.

In a regular menstrual cycle, the egg sits around in the uterus for a few days and then is dissolved into the endometrium. When this happens, a new stage in the cycle begins.

Now the uterus must renew its lining. Over the next two to seven days, the endometrium loosens and slips out of the uterus through the cervix, down the vagina and trickles out of our bodies. We call this time of flowing blood MENSTRUATION.

Menstrual "blood" is really a mixture of mucus and secretions from your vagina and cervix with the blood and mucus of the endometrium. The blood stains everything so it looks red, brown or pink, but, as you'll see, what comes out of your body during menstruation is stickier and thicker than blood. On that white pad or tampon, it sure looks like a lot! But really you only bleed about four to six tablespoons each period.

Even before your first period comes, though, you're bound to find some sticky white or clear stuff in your underwear. This DISCHARGE is mucus from your cervix and vagina and is perfectly natural. A woman's vagina produces mucus when she gets sexually excited and the mucus acts as lubricant during sexual penetration. But our bodies also produce these secretions every day to wash our internal organs, keeping them clean and free of infection. And just like everything else about human bodies, the amount of discharge varies from person to person — some women have more discharge than others.

Watch your discharge carefully so that you'll know what's normal for your body. It'll have a faint smell that's particular to you and will be clear or creamy white in colour, sometimes stringy and other times chunky, depending on where you are in your menstrual cycle. If your discharge is ever especially strong-smelling or an odd colour, or your vagina is itchy, it may mean that you have an infection and need to visit a doctor or health practitioner for a checkup.

Cycling: How Long? How Often?

Your "menstrual cycle" is the length of time it takes from the beginning of one period to the beginning of the next. Menstruation is often said to happen once every *month*, but this isn't always the case. The average cycle is about twenty-eight days, but this is just the *average*. It's just as normal to have twenty days between periods, or forty days. Some women never have a regular cycle: they'll have a period after twenty days and then they won't have another period for thirty days. Sometimes when a girl first starts menstruating, her period will come once and then not return for a few months or even a year.

Question: Do you all know when you'll get your
periods?
Susan: Not really, it varies.
Jeananne: Mine comes between the third and the
seventh of every month.
Maja: I don't know, mine's sort of whenever it
feels like coming, there it is.
Janti: Whenever there's something important
happening, I swear.
Susan: Yeah, that's when it is!
Janti: And every once in a while it comes right
before something big. Like school. This

year I finished it just before school started.
I'm like, "Yayyyy!"

Jeananne: I started the day school started.

Susan: I got it on a camping trip and I wasn't
supposed to get it on the camping trip.

Jeananne: Great.

Susan, Janti, Jeananne and Maja (13 – 14)

People also bleed for different lengths of time. For some women, the bleeding lasts only one or two days. For others, they can have a period that lasts for a week or more.

My mother thought I was pregnant once because my period didn't come for two months and then it lasted for two whole weeks when it finally came.

Claudia Marques (17)

If your period lasts longer than two weeks, you should talk to your mom and see a doctor. It may just be that your body is still figuring out how to menstruate; on the other hand, you might be sick and this is your body's way of telling you that there's a problem.

Where Babies Can Come In

If a woman has sexual intercourse, her monthly cycle of menstruation may be interrupted. During sexual intercourse, a woman guides a man's penis into her vagina. Liquid, called SEMEN, which is made up of millions of SPERM comes out of the man's penis. SPERM are the male version of a woman's egg. The sperm in the semen travel along the woman's vagina, through her cervix, uterus and into the fallopian tube. If the woman has recently ovulated, the man's semen and the woman's egg may meet up. The egg takes one sperm from the semen into itself and so becomes fertilized. The fertilized egg sticks to the endometrium, or blood lining, of the woman's uterus. It grows into an EMBRYO which matures into a FETUS, or baby. The blood lining protects and cradles the baby and as the baby grows, the uterus expands. This is the process of PREGNANCY.

When a woman is pregnant, monthly bleeding stops because the blood is needed inside the uterus to cushion the baby until it is born. Then a lot of blood comes out with the baby. After giving birth, a woman's menstrual cycle takes a few months to get back on track and will often return with a different pattern and with different signals and sensations. While a mother breastfeeds her baby, she probably will not menstruate.

> Of course, it kind of hits you sometimes, the shock of it that I can create another being. That was a big thing the first time I got my period. It was like, Wow! I could make another human being. With the help of someone else, of course, but that I can do this, I have the power to create. It's kind of a shocking thing, but a good thing.
>
> *Tiffanie Neilson (16)*

Sex: Proceed With Caution

Just because you may get your period at age twelve doesn't mean that your body is finished growing. Your breasts will get larger and your hips will continue to widen for the next couple of years. You'll also grow a little taller and even in your late teens you'll notice other signs of physical maturity too, like a change in your face's shape, more body hair and clearer skin.

Your body is maturing inside too. Your cervix and vagina will become thick and strong, and develop protective secretions. But your vagina, cervix and uterus still won't be fully mature until you're in your late teens and early twenties!

This is a very important thing to know if you're thinking of having sexual intercourse. Young women who have penetrative sex (where the penis goes into the vagina or anus) before their bodies are fully matured are far more likely to get sexually transmitted diseases (STDs), including HIV/AIDS. Signs of STD infection include unusual or heavy cramping. If you are sexually active and experience excessive cramping, be sure to talk to a doctor or health care practitioner.

Girls between the ages of fifteen to nineteen have some of the highest rates for STDs. This isn't because they're having tons of sex but because young women's sexual organs take a long time to reach full maturity and are vulnerable to disease until then.

Making the decision to have sex is a really serious one. Besides the worries of getting pregnant or catching life-threatening diseases, sex can stir up a lot of mixed emotions. Proceed with caution! If you or someone you know is planning on having sex, make sure that condoms and plenty of water-based lubricant — both are available at any drugstore — are used for your protection. Talk about your plans first, then take things slowly and be gentle so that your body has time to relax and to produce the helpful secretions that will act as a natural lubricant.

When Your Periods Stop

Sometimes a woman's periods will stop. Months may go by without any sign of blood. The fancy name for this disappearance is AMENORRHEA. Your cycle can stop for a number of different reasons.

If you have had sexual intercourse and your period has stopped, you may be pregnant. It's important to figure this out as soon as possible so that you have lots of time to plan ahead. You can easily and privately take a pregnancy test (the kits are available at drugstores) or visit a clinic or doctor. Being a pregnant teenager is a tough situation. Keep in mind that you have choices: you can have an abortion, give the baby up for adoption, or keep it. Be sure to think ahead to the future and talk with people who you are close to about your concerns and plans.

There are other reasons for the disappearance of menstruation. Some drugs, like the birth control pill, may cause menstruation to stop or the blood flow to become very light. Menstruation also stops when you have too little body fat because you've dieted too much. A sign of ANOREXIA (dieting until your body starts to starve to death) is amenorrhea. Fewer or shorter periods can be an early warning sign of anorexia. Extreme stress or illness can also stop your period.

If your period has disappeared, make sure that you get to the doctor to find out why. It may be because you're very stressed about school or it might be a serious health condition.

Menopause

Menstruation will stop forever when a woman reaches her early fifties. At this point, her body is no longer interested in having babies and her hormones slow down. This end of menstruation is called MENOPAUSE.

Menopause is like puberty in reverse. A menopausal woman's periods become irregular and eventually they stop completely. During this time, a woman may experience other things like sudden changes in body temperature (called "hot flashes"), mood swings and bursts of energy.

Menopause means a woman can no longer get pregnant but it doesn't mean the end of her sex life. After menopause some women feel very powerful and free, ready for the challenges of a new stage in life. Other women may be sad because they're no longer fertile and they may feel less feminine and attractive. Some women worry about their health because the hormones associated with menstruation make our bones strong and protect us from certain cancers. Most women feel a mixture of these things at menopause, just like the confusion a teenage girl may feel when she's going through puberty.

FIGURING THINGS OUT

❂

Signals: How to Tell When
Your Period's Coming

SOME WOMEN'S CYCLES never follow a predictable pattern. Teenagers might find this is especially true. You may be worried that at any moment you'll suddenly start to bleed right through your jeans!

However, your body usually gives you signals to let you know that the blood's on its way. You just have to figure out what these signals are. Every woman's menstrual signals are different and these signals change over time. Pay close attention to your body and your emotional ups-and-downs to learn what your signals are. Figuring out these signals will prepare you for your next menstrual period.

I've figured it out. I know about two days before when I'm going to have my period. It's not regular at all, but I can tell when it's coming. My wisdom teeth are growing in so my gums hurt and bleed two days before; then I'm bleeding from both ends! It's horrible,

I'm in so much pain! And then there's getting to sleep at night with the backache. And nothing works for it. I can be taking pain killers all day, but it's just this dull ache. The breast enlargement is a pain. It's like waking up some mornings and going, "Oh my god, I'm a size bigger! What the hell is this?"

Once my period begins the emotional ups-and-downs go away. My breasts go back to normal. As soon as my period starts, everything goes back to normal, but I still get that dull backache.

Tiffanie Neilson (16)

Here are some signals women experience a few days before the first day of bleeding. You may experience some of these sensations regularly when you menstruate, or you may experience none at all!

- lower backache

- vivid dreams

- feeling hyper and full of energy with little need for sleep

- feeling tired, sleeping a lot more than usual for a few days

- pimples

- intense sexual arousal (feeling horny)

- depression, sadness and crying for no reason

- clumsiness

- urinating more often

- diarrhea or constipation
- ESP — you just *know* who that is on the phone!
- change in appetite, cravings for particular kinds of food, especially chocolate!
- daydreaming, thoughtfulness, active imagination
- feeling like dancing, drawing, painting or writing poetry
- headaches and nausea
- bloating in the breasts, belly, feet and fingers
- cramps!
- assertiveness, aggressiveness, standing up for yourself and others
- temper tantrums
- giggling fits

You may discover a pattern to your behaviour and moods based on your cycle. The day before your period you might get angry easily, but when you're bleeding you may feel like writing poetry and dancing. Some women's monthly periods arrive at the same time as their best friends', their roommates' or their sisters'. Others discover that their cycles follow the phases of the moon. Understanding your period and seeing how it is with other women can give you a feeling of secret connection and mysterious power!

My last heavy period was in 1987 when I went to the Michigan Women's festival. My period wasn't even due. At one of the concerts the MC asked: "Who's menstruating?" About a third of the women hollered and put up their hands. Then she said, "Who didn't expect to menstruate?" About half of these women put up their hands. You get seven thousand women together and something weird happens.

Ruth Wood (50s)

Cramps

One of the most common complaints about menstruation has to do with cramps. DYSMENORRHEA is a very big word for these rotten pains in the lower abdomen. Cramps are natural things that happen to almost everyone at some time, although some women never have any pain at all. Cramps can come during or before the bleeding starts.

Susan: I'm glad I don't get really bad cramps because I know people who have to stay home because of them.

Jeananne: Cramps feel like I've been holding it in and not going to the bathroom for a really long time. It feels like bad gas and you want to let it out. But it won't come out.

Susan and Jeananne (13 & 14)

The key with menstrual cramps seems to be to get your body to relax. There are a lot of different ways to try to relax. Some will work better for you than others. However, sometimes it just seems impossible to unwind!

You have awful cramps right now. *What to do?*

- Go for a walk. Breathe deeply, feeling your chest fill with air. Look at the sights around you. Loosen your limbs. Stretch! Relax ....

- Aerobics anyone? Some women find that vigorous exercise is the best cure for cramps. It refreshes you — mind and body — and after, your muscles will naturally relax.

- Take a hot bath. Throw in some aromatherapy bath scents made especially for easing cramps. The heat of the water helps your body relax. A hot water bottle or a warm purring cat placed over your belly may also do the trick. (But don't take the cat in the bath tub!)

- Drink raspberry leaf tea. For some, this works like magic.

In the long term, there are other things you can do:

- Talk to your mom and other female relatives. Find out what they've done for cramps. What works for one family member might help another. Who knows what secrets Great Aunt Cecile has!

- What you eat affects your *whole* body. For some people, caffeine products like chocolate, cola, coffee and tea cause rotten cramps and lousy moods before their periods. Eat fruit and veggies instead of junk food and try to maintain a balanced diet.

- Exercise daily. Rollerblade, play tag football or hackey-sac, or walk the dog. We sometimes spend too much time indoors. There's a big beautiful world out there!

- Don't smoke. This nasty habit isn't just bad for your lungs, but also for your skin, gums and breath, and is related to menstrual cramping.

- Use the calendar at the back of this book to chart your periods. Try to see if there are any patterns to your pain, your diet, your activities and moods. Compare your cycle to your friends'.

- If your cramps are really awful, you feel faint, nauseous, have diarrhea or are throwing up and none of this stuff helps, talk to your doctor. There are pain-relieving drugs you can take, both prescription and those found on the shelf at the drugstore. Always ask your doctor or pharmacist what does and doesn't mix with any other drugs that you may be taking.

Period Positive!

Not all menstrual sensations are bad! Many women also feel more creative or energetic, caring or sexy around their periods. Your body may seem more sensitive and aware, and your senses especially sharp. During so much of our daily schedules, we often forget that we have bodies and spend too much time inside of our heads. Periods have a way of reminding us that our brain and our body are connected. When we remember this connection, the feeling of wholeness that we experience gives us a new and special way of looking at the world.

> After the first day of bleeding I feel a rush of energy —
> I feel like I can accomplish anything. I have come to
> appreciate this "second day strength" and I look for-
> ward to it because on that day anything is possible.
> *Carolyn Saunders (20s)*

Often we women are taught that menstruating is a nuisance and so we only notice the unpleasant aspects of it. Try hard to pay attention to the other experiences you have around your period. You may be pleasantly surprised!

Pads and Tampons

There are many different ways to take care of your menstrual blood. The two main ways are pads and tampons. You can buy both kinds of products in the grocery store or pharmacy. Some young women find it helpful to experiment with pads or tampons before their period begins so that they're prepared. It's a good idea to have some in your bathroom or purse or knapsack in case your period arrives unexpectedly. Other women often have pads or tampons with them and are always happy to share with someone in need. Don't be shy to ask — we all know what it feels like to be caught by surprise!

A tampon is a small length of compressed cotton with a

string attached to the end of it. You insert the tampon into your vagina with an applicator or your fingers so that just the string hangs out of your body. The cotton absorbs your menstrual blood and when it's full, you pull it out by the string and throw it away. It's *very important* not to leave the tampon inside your vagina for more than four hours at a time because a nasty bacteria can develop. This bacteria causes a rare but life-threatening illness called Toxic Shock Syndrome. Use the lightest absorbency of tampon that you can and switch to pads at night.

Each box of tampons contains instructions. When you first try to insert one, be sure you are in a space that gives you lots of room and privacy. Read the instructions carefully. When you insert the tampon, it's helpful to stand with one foot on the toilet seat lid or the edge of the bathtub because this opens up your vagina a little. Use a hand-held mirror to help find your vaginal opening and feel around gently with your fingers. It's essential that you put the tampon into your vagina, *not* into your anus, the hole between your buttocks. (See diagram page 28.) Using tampons requires some practice. It may take you a few tries to get the tampon in so that it feels comfortable.

> My most memorable period was the first time I ever used tampons. I was twelve and had had perhaps two or three periods. I was a member of a swim club and we were to participate in a swim meet over the weekend. I was excited but during a visit to the bathroom I discovered a brown stain in my panties. What a disaster! You couldn't go swimming if you had your period, I thought.

I couldn't face watching my teammates compete while I sat in the bleachers. I decided that the only way I would be able to carry on with the weekend was to use tampons. I went into the drugstore, bought the tampons and brought them back to my room. I locked myself in the bathroom and poured over the instructions. My mother claims I told her that, "I had a terrible time getting it in and afterwards I was all hot!"

No one knew about my secret that weekend. I swam with the rest of them. I even won a couple of ribbons. I am very proud of that weekend. Who says you can't go swimming when you have your period!

Debra Wiens (30s)

Some women feel more comfortable using pads. Pads are flat, compact layers of cotton that have a sticky strip on one side. The sticky side attaches to the crotch of your underwear and the pad catches your blood as it flows out of your vagina.

In my twenties I gave up tampons because I missed those cosy white cushions between my legs and the feeling of blood gently flowing out. I was also tired of struggles in cramped public washrooms, trying to find the damn string and trying to pull it at the right angle so that the bloated cotton ball would come out easily.

Yolande Bélanger Mennie (30s)

Just like tampons, pads should be changed every few hours. Store-bought pads are thrown away after each use, but some women make their own cloth pads and wash them so that they can be reused for their next cycle. For more information on cloth pads and other options, see pages 129-130.

Keeping Track

When I first came to Canada, it was really hard. I had no friends. Everybody knew how to speak English but me. I started right into school, into grade eight. I got a lot of pressure from other kids to do things. I wanted to be cool, so I got into drugs and smoking. Then I got into trouble from my parents who said they would move us back to Portugal if I didn't stop. My marks at school were bad. I wanted more freedom but my father wouldn't let me go out and we fought a lot. This went on for about three years. It was a very bad experience.

During this time, my periods were so painful. Oh my god, it was awful! At first I didn't realize that my painful periods had to do with stress. Then I started enjoying more sports and left behind the bad crowd. The sports helped a bit. Then I started getting counselling and that really helped too. With that I had an agenda and I had to mark every month when my period came. After a while I started to notice the pattern. I looked at my past agenda and saw that I would cry almost every day and be stressed out. On the new agenda everything was good. I compared them and saw how different they were.

Claudia Marques (17)

If you keep track of your menstruation times, you can learn a lot about your general health. At the back of this book there's a twelve month calendar. When you have your period, mark each bleeding day on the calendar. After a few bleeding cycles you may begin to see a pattern, say that your period comes about every thirty-two days or maybe that it always comes near the end of every month. This will help you to predict when your next period is due. However, some women's menstrual cycles are very irregular — especially when they first start menstruating. They may not have a period for months at a time. It's important to learn what is natural and normal for *you*. If your period's late or your cycle develops an irregularity, this might mean that something's up: Are you under a lot of stress and need to relax? Are you getting enough rest, exercise and food? Are you pregnant? Your menstrual cycle is like an internal doctor who gives you health reports throughout the month.

CELEBRATIONS

◎

"Why Now?"

SOME GIRLS WONDER WHY they have to menstruate when they have no plans of having babies for many years. But being a woman is about much more than being able to have babies. Menstruation tells you a lot of important information about your body's health and can reflect how you're feeling about life. Menstruation says to the world that you're becoming an adult and deserve the rights and responsibilities of adulthood. Menstruation reminds us that we are connected to the world around us, that we have rhythms like the ocean tides and cycles like the moon. And menstruation also connects us to other women.

> Since I was the first girl in my grade to have the honour of going through menstruation, I was entirely alone in my feelings. I tried desperately to keep it a secret. Then one day that summer I received a phone call from my best friend. Her first four simple yet wonderful words filled me with absolute joy: "I got my period." I rushed over to her house to compare menstrual cramps. We complained happily of the burden we had to go through each month and we pitied the

poor girls who had not yet reached our level of maturity. That fall we returned to school with an air of superiority, for we were now women!

Brandy Ford (19)

First Time Parties

MENARCHE (men-ark-ie), the fancy name for first menstruation, has been celebrated in some cultures with special traditions and parties. It's understood to mean that a child has become an adult, a girl has become a woman, and that this change deserves special recognition.

Different cultures have various ways of marking a girl's menarche. In some Jewish families, a young woman gets a very light slap on the cheek when she has her first period. Some people think that this tradition happens because the young woman must take notice that she is no longer a child under her parents' control while others say that it's a way of scaring away bad spirits. The Asante people of Ghana celebrate a girl's first menstruation with a party in her honour. She's treated like royalty, given gifts and there's lots of singing and dancing to celebrate. The !Gwi of southern Africa celebrate menarche by decorating the body of the young woman, and her husband, with intricate patterns.

In the past, the Yurok people of California believed that a menstruating woman should be separated from the other members of the community since she had such incredible powers. It was thought that the bleeding time should not be used for daily living, but for prayers and worship. At menarche a girl was taken to a menstrual shelter where she performed secret rites and took a special bath. She was given special clothes and ate only certain foods. Though this practice is no longer common, some Yurok women are careful to keep their tradition alive.

The Oglala Sioux people of the North American prairies have a long history of revering the menstruating woman as a powerful being. The newly menstruating girl would traditionally undergo a purification ritual and undertake instruction from a holy woman. She would be compared to the sacred Mother Earth, yet her power was also considered to be dangerous if the proper rituals and instructions were not given. But once these conditions were met, her holiness was considered to extend to the entire tribe, not just to herself. After these rituals, the young woman was told: "You are the tree of life. You will now be pure and holy, and may your generations to come be fruitful! Wherever your feet touch will be a sacred place, for now you will always carry with you a very great influence."*

*Serenity Young, *An Anthology of Sacred Texts By and About Women*. New York: Crossroad, 1993. Page 231.

Bleeding Power

Cultures all over the world have special rules and rituals for the menstruating woman.

Some cultures believe menstruation is very important and so celebrate menstruation to make it a special, sacred time. Other cultures are afraid of the power of menstruation and consider it dangerous. They try to control a menstruating woman by preventing her from doing many things, like taking part in certain religious or recreational events. This is what is called a menstrual "taboo."

Most often cultures have *both* celebrations and taboos for menstruation. This shows that, no matter what their views, people all over the world believe that menstruation is *very powerful*. But it's confusing to try and understand how people view the power of menstruation. Sometimes this power is considered both good and bad at the same time.

Many cultures have rules that prevent women from having sex, working or cooking during menstruation. This sounds like a menstrual taboo, but this is also a way for a woman to take a holiday every month. In some societies menstruating women must stay in special "menstrual huts" that are separated from the rest of the community. Some women find that this restricts their freedom because they can't leave this area. Other women find it a good place to relax and talk with women friends, or a place where they can enjoy some privacy, do creative projects or say special prayers. How would *you* feel about this?

Lots of societies believe menstrual blood has magical properties. In some cultures menstrual blood is used by a wife to make sure her husband is not attracted to other women, while in others, a man uses it to make sure his wife isn't attracted to other men! Menstrual blood has also been used as a poison against enemies or as a protector from evil forces. People have believed that menstrual blood can cure a number of severe medical conditions. One of the most common beliefs about menstrual blood is that it has life-giving power. Many societies have special "fertility" rituals that use menstrual blood to help women have healthy babies and to help fields grow good crops.

It's easy to think that our society has no menstrual taboos or rituals and that we don't think menstrual blood is magical. But is that really true? How do people react when they see someone else's menstrual blood? If they act in some extreme fashion, this probably means they feel menstrual blood has a certain kind of power.

Here are some examples of menstrual rules and rituals from around the world and from different times in history:

- The Kaska of western Canada and the Warao of Venezuela created special "menstrual huts" for their menstruating women.

- In ancient Rome, it was commonly believed that menstrual blood could cure certain illnesses. In Morocco at the beginning of this century, people believed it could cure wounds and open sores.

- Some cultures, like North American whites, call menstruation a "curse." Other people, like the Ebrié of the Ivory Coast in Africa, think it's a curse if a young woman should *lose* her periods.

- Many cultures, like the Asante of Ghana, have special parties to celebrate the powers of the menstruating woman. But there are also other cultures, like the Greek Orthodox church, which prevent menstruating women from taking part in religious ceremonies like the communion.

- The Mae Enga of New Guinea used menstrual blood as a poison against enemies, while the Asante in Ghana and the Kwakiutl of the Pacific Northwest use menstrual blood as a way of protecting themselves from evil forces.

- In many hunting cultures, menstruating women are not allowed to touch the hunting equipment before a big hunt. Some agricultural communities, however, use menstrual blood to bless their crops.

- The women of the Rungus of Borneo let their blood flow freely during menstruation. They don't use a menstrual product to absorb their blood, but spend their bleeding time sitting on specially dried moss or bamboo slats. When they wish to move around or change positions, they rinse themselves and the moss or slats with water.

- The Beng women of the Ivory Coast spend their menstrual time preparing a meal that's considered a delicacy and takes many hours to prepare. This dish is eaten only by menstruating women and their close female friends.

• Some scholars believe that all religious celebrations and rituals first began with the celebration of menstruation. Menstrual blood was considered by ancient cultures to be one of the most sacred substances since it, like the blood of childbirth, is the only kind of blood that's not linked with death and dying — but with the potential for new life. The root word for "ritual" comes from a Sanskrit word that means "menses." This links menstruation with the very origins of religious rituals.

Celebrate Your Sweet Secret

What's your tradition? How would *you* like to celebrate menarche? Here are some suggestions:

• Get something special for yourself the day you have your very first period, like a new book or flowers from your neighbour's garden. Give something special to your friends and sisters when they have their first periods.

• Have a Period Party — girls only — and eat strawberries, tomatoes and red licorice.

• Wear something red on the first day of your period every month — no one but you will ever know!

• Dunk tampons in water glasses to test their absorbency.

- Explain menstruation to your baby brother and make sure he appreciates the importance of it.

- Keep a period diary and compare your menstrual cycle to the phases of the moon.

- Hang out with Mom and try treating her like the adult she can be.

- Do something that makes you feel powerful and strong every time you have your period.

Meeting the Challenge

Just as views of menstruation change from culture to culture, many things about menstruation itself vary from woman to woman: the length of bleeding time, the amount of blood and what you use to catch it, the sensations you feel and how regularly your bleeding happens. These characteristics also change over time. You can expect your menstrual story to transform slightly throughout your lifetime just as your personality grows stronger and your tastes and opinions develop. That's all part of growing up and becoming an individual, strong and separate from your family and friends, yet linked to them through love and shared experiences.

A long time ago, in my Haida culture, my people used to believe that menstruating women had powers. The women in my society were revered and respected. Women were looked to as the backbone of our society.

Every month, menstruating women would go to menstruating huts and these women shared songs and stories with one another. And when a young woman started her periods, a big potlatch was held in her honour. The whole village would participate. There would be feasting, songs, dances; gifts were given. All of this was done just for her.

Roberta Kennedy (30s)

Most cultures now no longer celebrate menstruation as the beginning of womanhood. Without these celebrations it's sometimes hard to know what a beautiful and powerful thing it is to become a woman.

You should be proud of your body and respect it by getting to know how it works. When your period comes, mark it on the calendar and see how many days it takes for your next period to come. Try keeping a diary and note how your body feels during different times in your cycle.

But most importantly, *talk with the important women in your life*, listen to their stories and share your own. Tell them about all of the changes in your body and they will tell you of the changes they have experienced in their lives. You may be surprised to find that many will understand your mixed feelings of pride and fear, shame and excitement at growing up a woman.

Becoming a woman is a challenge, but your body knows you're up to it!

More Menstruation Facts ... and Where to Find Them

MENSTRUATION

STORIES

☉

*H*AVE YOU EVER HELD A SEASHELL to your ear and listened to the whistling sound that comes from deep inside its pink spiral? Closed your eyes and *just listened,* barely breathing, to the story it has to tell? Sometimes that quiet waiting, that still-easy feeling is just what you need to catch up with yourself, to hear your heart beat and feel the sympathetic rhythm of the air rising and falling deep inside your belly.

This is the sweet secret of the shell. It lures you to come and discover the sea, but takes you to yourself instead.

Listening to another person's secrets and stories — like putting your ear against the cool lip of the seashell — is sometimes the only way to really understand what's happening in your own life. You probably already know that when you listen closely to stories from your mom, aunts, sisters and friends, you learn new and important information about your favourite people. But now and then you also discover *something else* in their stories, something familiar — a piece of your life in someone else's story. And you can even hear these echoes from your life in a *stranger's* story.

Sometimes this thought or experience that you share with another person is so surprising that it sends a shiver down your backbone like a bolt of lightning! More often it is a warm feeling of recognition, since what you learn about yourself from the story of another is always something you already know deep inside of yourself. But it just needs the words of another, like the echo of the seashell, to draw it to the surface and make itself known.

The women who wrote the stories that follow talk about the many different feelings young women have around the time of their first period. You may find yourself in some of these stories, or you may hear the voices of other women you know. And later you will get to tell *your* story to the people around you — your friends, your sisters, your mom. They'll learn about you and they may even learn something new about themselves. *Together* — telling our stories, listening and learning — this is how we women come to understand the secrets of our bodies.

WAITING

These stories describe some of the different feelings and thoughts young women have about getting their first periods. Waiting for your first period can be a strange time. Some girls are the first in their group of friends to have it while others wait and wait. You may look forward to menstruation with excitement or you might be afraid, or maybe you will feel a bit of both. Thinking about this new experience gives you a chance to plan and prepare for it.

Blood

JANE EATON HAMILTON

*Melly and Joyce are on period patrol. Jane Eaton
Hamilton tells the story of Melly and her best friend
Joyce, who check their underwear "six hundred times a
day" to see if they've started bleeding yet. Melly and Joyce
have got menstruation on the brain ....*

THEY GIVE US ALL IQ TESTS and shoot us into a special class,
all the nerds and geeks and wild girls with brains. We do
stuff like watch TV and play chess and study dead poets and
make a graffiti mural on a gym wall and bus to the city to
visit art museums and junk like that. Everybody hates us and
we hate them so it works out. We put on *The Merchant of
Venice*. I try out to be Portia and just really see myself as
Portia only I don't get the part, this stuck-up dork named
Michelle does. Like I'll ever act again, I'm so humiliated.

One day we're all outside playing baseball for compulsory
PE and my friend Joyce and I say can we go inside to Mrs
Nacho and she says Yeah which is why we call her Mrs Nacho
she's not too bright. Joyce and me use the can, looking for

blood in our panties. We do this six hundred times a day because only Sonia Cole's got it and we want it and we wear bras so it's about time. Sonia Cole is tall like an apartment building and has a stubby face and long straight brown hair down to her waist.

Joyce and me wander into the classroom, not wanting to go back outside. Between Doug Baxter's desk and Joanne Phillip's desk are four drops of blood on the tile in a little line one two three four not smeared. I look at Joyce and she looks at me with her peculiar eyes (her mother is Norwegian) and we go Oh my god and squeal and jump up and down and hold our crotches. Because Sonia Cole was in the can, she left the baseball field five minutes before we did and went back because she's pitcher and likes balls flying through the air at her, she's nuts.

So here we are it's June and there's blood on the classroom floor. I stick out my foot and push my toe at one of the blood blobs. Joyce goes Oh oh oh you're so gross. I get blood on my sneaker and Joyce's face goes red and she claps her hands she's so excited. I stick my toe up and go Yah yah yah I'm going to get you with Sonia Cole's blood, I'm going to get you.

Joyce goes, Yuck, ew, Melly you're so disgusting. I go Ho ho ho and she starts giggling and we hold our stomachs and totter around the back of the classroom laughing so hard it hurts.

Then, Joyce goes quiet and even her sunburn slides off her face, she's white as a tampon. She looks around to make sure we're alone. She got felt up by Steve Harvey — what if he heard us? She whispers Melly Melly we got to clean it up.

I realize she's right, it's Sonia Cole's blood. On the floor there's three red dots and one snaky line and I have Sonia Cole's menstrual blood on my shoe and what if Steve Harvey really did come in? I would like to kiss him, don't tell Joyce. I would like to go to third base under the weeping willow tree behind my house and he would say Melly your boobs are bigger than Joyce's Melly touch me down there which is where the sun doesn't like to shine except in nudist camps where my Aunt Rita goes.

So I go, Like, with what?

Joyce looks out the window and says Geez Melly I think the game's stopping think of something we can't just leave it there.

We both stare at Sonia Cole's blood which is red as lipstick. The sun's coming in and making it sparkle. Joyce moans and says What are we going to do Melly?

And I go I don't know.

Joyce goes, The girls' washroom! We'll get some paper towel and get it wet and clean it up.

You go, I tell her.

No you, she says.

You first, I say. We run through the hall on our tiptoes and I get the paper towel and stand on the ring under the sink that's five feet wide and the fountain starts up and I stick the paper under while Joyce watches the hall to make sure no one's coming. We sneak back to the classroom leaving water drips all the way.

Shh, Joyce goes and giggles.

Shh yourself, I go.

We pull open the classroom door and walk in so slow this must be a math test. Which actually we don't have, they don't grade us because we have genius IQs we're very smart. We just get comments: I don't feel Melanie is working up to her true potential, I believe Joyce's attention is wavering.

Are you having problems at home, dear? Mrs Nacho asked me once after I fell asleep during science. No ma'am my hamster died and I'm so sad. No ma'am I was up all night menstruating.

The blood's still there and outside we hear shouts and voices getting near and Joyce looks at me and I shove the paper towel at her and she rips it in two and shoves half back. We don't say a thing. We breathe heavy. We get down on the floor and twitch and finally stick out our soggy paper towels and do it quick, one two, the way our mothers taught us to wipe counters and it's gone.

But then we jump out of our skins screaming and Joyce knocks into Joanne's desk and her *Norton's English Literature* goes thud on the floor and I throw my towel as fast as I can towards the garbage bin. It's Owen Carmichael, the fat kid, in his fat boy's white shorts with his pudgy legs and his turned-down white ankle socks and his belly. Plus zits all over his face.

What're you doing, he says.

Nothing, Joyce goes, we weren't doing anything what's wrong with you?

I had a nosebleed, Owen says. He holds out a bloody Kleenex.

So Joyce looks at me and I look at Joyce like, This is too rude. Everyone else comes in behind Owen and we all sit down and then we do fractions.

WHAT TO DO ...

... with used pads when you're visiting a friend's house?

Put it in the garbage. There's no need to be ashamed: bleeding is natural! However, you may feel more comfortable if you fold the used pad in half and wrap it in some toilet paper before putting it in the garbage. Don't try to flush it down the toilet!

... when you get bloodstains on your underwear or pants?

Rinse the garment in cold water. If it's still stained, apply laundry soap to the stain, scrub lightly and soak it for a few hours in warm water. Rinse well.

... when you get your period but don't have a pad or tampon handy?

Toilet paper or facial tissue stuffed in your underwear should hold you over for a bit. Unfortunately, since it's not pinned down, the paper may slide out of place. If you're at home, you can pin an old facecloth to your underwear until you can get to a store. If you're in a public place, ask another woman for help. Every woman has been in "menstrual need" at least once in her life and chances are she'll be more than happy to do what she can.

The Summer
I was Ten

ARDELLE STEUERNOL

*In "The Summer I was Ten," Ardelle Steuernol
remembers the time when her two best friends already
had their periods but she didn't yet have hers.
Her friends' special code names for menstruation, like
"Aunt Rose" and "monthlies," add to the mystery.
To the ten year old Ardelle, having your period means
being part of a very important club. And it's a club that
Ardelle desperately wants to join!*

THE SUMMER I WAS TEN I hung around the farm and kept a close surveillance on my underwear. Helen and Thelma, my best friends, lived three miles down the concession road. They were two years older than me and when they started to menstruate within weeks of each other, I felt excluded. They talked about their *monthly* when we were alone and carried on private conversations in the schoolyard when there were no boys around.

"Aunt Rose came to visit this morning," one would remark.

"Is she staying long?" the other would question.

"About a week," the first would reply and they would cover their mouths with their hands and giggle.

When Helen and Thelma invited me to bicycle the three miles to their houses for an afternoon, I made some excuse and stayed at home, alone.

Mother was delighted with my sudden interest in the domestic side of family life and proceeded to teach me the art of cooking. I was making elderberry and apple pies, one after the other, when I noticed a red stain on the front of my jeans. I yanked open the elastic in my panties and there it was — the spot I had been waiting for!

Mother was picking apples in the orchard and had missed this historic event. "It happened!" I shouted, running out of the house, letting the screen door slam behind me. "Mom, I've got my monthly!" The button and zipper of my jeans still hung open.

"Wait until I'm finished here and I'll get you a belt and pad," Mother answered.

Wait! How could I wait? I still had a three mile bicycle ride ahead of me if I was going to get this news to Helen and Thelma today. I imagined myself sitting tight on my bicycle seat so my new pad wouldn't slip. Maybe I would take an extra pad with me in case I had to change while I was there.

"Aunt Rose came today, " I would calmly announce to Helen and Thelma and then I would ask where to put the used pad after I had wrapped it in a tight bundle of toilet tissue.

Mother appeared to be moving in slow motion. I couldn't wait any longer.

"I'll show you now!" I yelled. I hooked my thumb under the elastic of my panties and pulled them away from my body.

"Oh!" Mother exclaimed, staring at the round red stain sitting about two inches below my belly button. "I think it's a false alarm dear," she said, picking the squashed elderberry off my panties.

BLOATING

Bloating is a condition that's caused by *water retention*. Before your period, hormone changes may cause your body to hold back some of the water you would usually pee or sweat out. If you're bloated, your breasts may be larger and tender, your pants may be tighter than usual around the waist and rings may not fit on your fingers. Even your feet can bloat! To keep bloating down, limit how much salty food you eat. Salt makes your body retain water and if you cut back on salt, your body will naturally release water.

THE PYRAMID

STEPHANIE STEARN

Stephanie Stearn, the author of this story, knows that not everyone wants to get their first period. Feeling frightened or just not interested in menstruation is quite normal too! Emily, the main character in "The Pyramid," is afraid that getting her period will change her forever. Emily likes who she is now and wants to stay the same always.

JUDY GOT HER PERIOD. My mother was on the phone with her mother and her mother told mine.

"Poor thing," I heard my mother say. "Is she all right?"

I went up to my room where I was building a tin can pyramid out of discarded pop cans that I'd found in the street. They were mostly green and red, but some were so filthy they almost lacked colour. I fished a few new ones out of my spring jacket. I had just positioned them at the top when I heard my mother's weight on the stairs. My door was shut with a warning hanging on the doorknob: DO NOT

DISTURB. I never turned it around to the other side that said MAID PLEASE MAKE UP ROOM — my mother didn't appreciate it.

"Emily?" she said through the door. I didn't answer right away. I was busy deciding whether or not to throw away the mud-tainted cans. They didn't look as nice as the shiny ones that I had drained myself.

"Can I come in?" she asked.

"Sure," I said. My mother came in, looked at me, then looked at the pyramid which at that point stood a good five feet tall.

"That was Judy's mother on the phone," she said.

"I know. I heard you."

"Judy has started her menstrual period," my mother said, still looking at the pyramid. "She's becoming a woman."

This made me laugh: Judy, not my closest friend, but the third on my list; the uncool Judy with her greasy bangs and long stringy hair; Judy with her tinsel teeth, rickety thin stick-body and cheerleader dreams; Judy, becoming a woman.

"What's so funny?" asked my mother.

"Nothing."

"Really, Emily, you always manage to make things so bloody difficult."

"What?"

My mother didn't answer. She seemed very interested in the pyramid, which was unusual, unless she was about to say what she always said when she came into my room: Why did

I collect junk and when exactly would I be throwing it out? Her silence had me on edge. I was used to predicting the actions of my family. I thought I had better help her along.

"Is there something wrong?" I asked.

"Do you know what menstruation is?"

"Sure," I lied.

"Who told you?" she asked, surprised.

"We took it in school."

"I don't think so," she said, relaxing. "Who told you?"

"Fleur Bradley," I said simply. I didn't like to admit that I didn't know something. I had an idea that it had something to do with bras and napkins or boys and make-up which was all that Fleur ever talked about any more. Something had happened to Fleur and I didn't like it. I stopped listening to her. She had slid from number two to number six on my friendship list.

"Well," my mother sighed. "What do you know?"

My face got red. I was a bad liar.

"Well?" she asked, knowing.

"I don't know."

"Poor Emily," she said. "I'd better tell you then since it could happen to you any day now."

"What?" I asked, horrified. She sat on my bed. I remained standing with my arms folded.

"Well ... all women ... all girls are capable of having a baby when they get to a certain age. When they get to this age, they start to bleed every month, and ..."

"I won't," I protested. But somehow I knew there were

no exceptions. I started to cry. My mother put her arms around me and tried to tell me what a wonderful privilege it was to be able to bleed every month.

The following Sunday, I was at Judy's house watching TV. The afternoon movie was *Whatever Happened to Baby Jane?* As the film progressed, I sat on the floor clutching an over-sized pillow to my stomach, fascinated. When I had to turn away, at the rat part, I saw that Judy was asleep on the couch. It figured that she would fall asleep while watching such a cool movie. She was still the same. It was a relief.

Blood and Chestnuts

KATHLEEN O'GRADY

*In this story, Kathleen O'Grady remembers what it was
like to be twelve and fascinated with the idea of having
a period. She can't understand why all of her friends
aren't as nosey about periods as she is: she wants to know
why women bleed, and how it looks and feels.
Mostly she can't wait to have a period of her own.
But when her first period begins, it's not
exactly what Kathy had been expecting.*

I USED TO THINK a lot about blood — about bleeding, really.
I spent my twelve year old days dreaming about it. I
would imagine walking slowly forward, in a school washroom full of watchful eyes, some malevolent, some congratu-
latory, as I released the dime that had been trapped forever in
my more-than-sweaty palm. My right hand would reach
forth with mechanical perfection to grasp the dime from my

left hand, forcefully pinching it between my index finger and thumb — I must not let it drop! My right arm would reach up and out in crane-like gestures until — *clink* — the dime was swallowed by the machine — and *clunk* — it issued forth a box weighted with necessity: mission completed.

I used to have this daydream repeatedly, varying only the character of watchful eyes, but never the movements. It was an elaborately planned procession for purchasing my first *sanitary napkin,* or, as I called it then in short bursts of consonantal force: *pad.*

My (hoped-for) day of purchase, I assured myself, would be accomplished markedly different from the processions of others who walked boastfully toward the machine, when really, we all heard from Elka's older sister that Terry and Lisa and Lori didn't need the gifts it bestowed. It was just a play put on for an eager but all-knowing audience.

My body had already started to create breasts for me; "like chestnuts," my friend Mary used to say. We would talk about them, but I never much cared for my "chestnuts." They were cumbersome, though I had not yet been plagued by a bra (or a "braazeeeere" as my mother would say in a painfully long and careful manner — "You'll soon have to wear a braazeeeere"). At recess the boys would target all the bra-wearers and snap the back strap. I was embarrassed for them at the sound it made.

Stephanie was the only one who really had her period. We were all in awe. We talked about getting ours and crowded her with questions: "Does it hurt?", "Do you feel

different?", "What does it *look* like?" We once tried to get
her to show us one of her used pads — just to see — but
she would have nothing of it. I don't remember her being
boastful or proud, but *we* were for her. We sort of had this
undiscussed competition to see who would be next. We
checked our underwear constantly and complained about
cramps we never had.

I was the one who asked the question "What does it *look*
like?" the most. I tried to think of an example (after the
failed attempt at asking Stephanie to see one of her pads) of
what the blood might look like, since it came out of such an
odd place. I would ask Stephanie, "Is it like when you cut
your hand? Like the time my mom cut her thumb with a
knife and it went way down deep and the blood was really
gross?" or "Is it like when the leaves fall and it rains and the
leaves bleed into the pavement?" None of these examples
(and countless more I used to think up) ever came close.
Once though, when they were teasing me about my "chestnuts," Stephanie said, "Yeah! The blood is like the colour of
chestnuts, not like *your* chestnuts, but *real* chestnuts." I
could never imagine this.

It was quite a few months before another one of us had
blood-stories to tell and Fate had slotted me next on the
blood-list. It may sound like a touch of corny drama, but I
had my first period December 28th, on the morning of my
thirteenth birthday.

I remember this morning very well. I had just gotten up
to go to the bathroom, still groggy with morning sleep, when

I perched myself on the toilet. My underwear was brown. I looked at it, disgusted, thinking that perhaps I had had an "accident" and had gone to the toilet in my sleep or something. But then as I wiped myself clean I suddenly realized that it was my *blood* that had caused the stain. I quickly shifted from disgust to jubilation. I thought of deep, ruddy brown chestnuts and the colour of my blood was remarkably close.

Then I made my mark in family history by waking my aunt Dee and everyone else within a hundred-mile radius. Aunt Dee was sleeping in my parents' room (staying over for Christmas vacation) when I yelled from the bathroom toward my mom's room, "MOM, MOM, GUESS WHAT?! I GOT MY PERIOD!!!" I had forgotten that my aunt and uncle were in my parents' bedroom. My aunt still tells everyone this story. That day I couldn't understand what she had found so funny about the mix-up, though I see the humour now.

I finally made my way to the guest room and told my mom about the discovery. She said, "Sssssshhhh. You'll wake the whole house. You know where I keep the *stuff* in the bathroom" — I distinctly recall her saying *stuff* like it was a first-aid kit I was to look for — "help yourself to it." I was disappointed. That was it. She was almost sad and a bit embarrassed that I was finally bleeding. I guess she was sorry to share with me what she considered a loss. I, on the other hand, saw it as a gain. She discussed it no further that day except in stifled laughs when my aunt Dee told her how she had been awakened that morning.

◎ Waiting ◎

I don't remember much else. I don't remember telling my friends about it, though I guess I called them right away. I never did perform my purchase in the school bathroom and I don't remember revelling in "blood and chestnut" talks any more. I suppose the novelty wore off.

I do remember Mary's period. She was number four, I think, by then. When she told her mother, her mother presented her with a pair of earrings, as if she had passed some sort of test. I was jealous. Mary thought the gift was a silly idea. Her mother was the only one who had done that. I told my mother about the earrings and I remember Mom telling me how silly it was. She thought it ridiculous, really. Of course I decided it was silly too. But in truth I wanted the earrings that Mary was embarrassed by.

Perhaps I've made my mother the ogre in this tale. This is not the case. She was always very open to my questions and encouraged my interest. I guess when all this happened, I was young and she was old, and it was one time when the gap couldn't be bridged.

Now my monthly bleeding is mostly a nuisance, though I sometimes romanticize about it. One time, in a Native Studies class in second year university, a shaman came in and was going to show some of his equipment to the class, but said he could not because there was a menstruating woman in the room. That bleeding woman was me. I was proud of it. It made me feel powerful. Another time I noticed that my monthly bleeding almost always came when there was a full moon. Again this gave me a sense of power, but a power of belonging to something beyond me. Now I take the birth control pill. This means my bleeding can be charted with exact accuracy on the calendar. This also means I no longer bleed at full moon — technology is now revoking my right to take part in the natural cycles of the world.

As I grow older, I no longer think of bleeding often. Sometimes though, in the fall, when I see leaf blood on the sidewalks and chestnuts on the ground, I think of Stephanie and Mary and the rest, and remember our early period talks with a warm fondness that never fails to make me smile.

WHAT'S PMS?

PMS stands for **pre-menstrual** syndrome. A "syndrome" is a bunch of health signals that alert you to the changes taking place in your body. Signs of PMS come on the days or weeks before a woman gets her menstrual period and ends when she starts bleeding.

Not all women experience PMS although many may sometimes feel a few of the signs associated with PMS. And not everyone can agree about what PMS is. We also aren't sure what it's caused by.

(cont'd)

However, most people agree that when a woman is experiencing PMS, she feels awful. Some PMS symptoms include very painful cramps, backaches, headaches and/or stomachaches, mood swings, dizziness and feeling very tired.

If you feel many of the PMS symptoms, you may want to talk about this with your parents, doctor or health care practitioner. There are lots of things they can do to help you if they are mature enough to understand how much pain you're in. You also may want to get in tune with your menstrual cycle by charting its pattern on a special calendar. Watch your diet, making sure you eat less salty and sweet foods, drink less cola and coffee, and don't smoke, because these things seem to make PMS worse. Reduce the stress in your life by exercising daily, getting plenty of sleep and taking time to relax. Try to express your feelings, particularly your angry ones more openly — don't let all this negative stuff stay bottled up inside you. Some women find that if they leave their feelings unexpressed, their PMS is more difficult.

THE ARRIVAL

When your first period happens, you can't believe it.
Even if you have learned all about menstruation and feel
prepared, it's still so surprising. You wonder,
"Is this really happening to me?"

Some girls don't learn much about menstruation so when
their periods arrive, they're shocked, even frightened or
angry. Others know to expect their periods but may be
surprised by their feelings or the responses of the people
around them. Either way, the day of your first period is a
special one. You'll remember this moment forever.

THE LOOK

SUE OSWALD

*Sue Oswald was born with multiple birth defects which
meant that she was hospitalized many times as a child.
In this story, she tells us what her life was like when she
was eleven years old and had severe scoliosis,
or curvature of the spine. For treatment of the scoliosis,
Sue has to lie flat on her back in a body cast for many
months in hospital and later at home. But Sue's medical
problems don't make her feel special or different. She
knows that, like any other girl her age, her body has a
lot of surprises to offer, and she's ready for each and every
one of them. Except, of course, for the pimples....*

I STARTED MY PERIOD flat on my back, in a body cast.

I spent the summer of 1972 in the hospital, in traction,
confined with fourteen girls in varying stages of hormonal
rage, and so learned to view the workings of the human
female body with a cool detachment.

The idea was to straighten the spine before the operation

and then keep it straight during growth. *Like Mom's tomato plants,* I thought. I remembered how my mother had tended her scoliotic stalks, how, despite daily watering and feeding, they fell down anyway. How she'd driven stakes into the ground, raised the sagging vines, and tied them to the posts for support until they were ready to be plucked.

So.

I looked in the mirror.

There would be traction, then an operation, then months at home in bed in a body cast. That made sense.

But this? What were these ugly, full whiteheads doing here? There. On my face?

"They're gross," I reported to my mother. "They make me look different."

"Not very different."

"Different enough."

In traction you lie there flat on your back, unable to move your head or legs, staring at the ceiling. "Prism glasses" help break the tedium.

Prisms are pyramid-shaped pieces of glass. When glued to a special frame, they become a unique kind of eyeglasses that let you *see down.* That's right. With the prism glasses resting across the bridge of your nose, you can see what's in front of you, such as a book propped open on your chest, or a letter you're writing on the TV tray. You can read without tiring your arms, or watch TV without straining your eyeballs. Or you can follow the snippets of activity that pass through the narrow lane of vision at the foot of the bed. All this while staring towards the ceiling.

Sometimes, when the light hits the prisms just right, a rainbow streaks across the line of vision — a burst of colour unexpected and welcome.

"Look at the rainbow!" I blurted one day to no one in particular.

"That's Roygeebiv," an anonymous voice responded. I couldn't place the voice, and whoever was talking was beyond my peripheral vision. "Who — ?"

"Roy G. Biv. The colours of the rainbow," The Voice responded, having obviously misunderstood.

"I don't get it."

"Tell me what colours you see," The Voice said.

"Red, orange, yellow — "

"Go on."

"Green, blue ... uh ... purple?"

"Indigo and violet."

"Ah. Indigo and violet."

"That's right. Indigo, violet."

"Roy G. Biv. It's an easy way to remember the colours of the rainbow, also known as the spectrum."

"The spectrum."

"The thing about rainbows is that they show up when you least expect them to."

Cheryl played records and talked too much. She'd wander around the ward blathering nonsense or reciting the words to the blasted Danny Kaye record she'd worn a groove in. She played the yellow record over and over on her cheap record player. She'd taped a penny on the arm to keep it from skipping.

"I'm late," the raspy voice recited. "I'm late — " *scratch scratch.*

On and on it went.

"No time to say —" *scratch scratch* "hello, goodbye —" *scratch scratch.*

Cheryl was older than the rest of us, but smaller, and especially small for her age. She'd float through the ward like an injured fairy, her blond hair and papery skin a wan reflection in the prisms. "I'm late —" she'd chant along with the record, skips and all, "I'm late —"

Late for *what* date? I wondered.

"Do you *mind*?" Denise yelled at Cheryl one night.

"No," Cheryl replied seriously. "Why should I mind?" Cheryl had played the stupid song over and over all day long and now was muttering it while everyone was trying to get to sleep. She wasn't really singing, or humming, or even talking. Just making noise.

"Tomorrow's a big day for me," Denise snapped again.

Denise was a biter. Normally she would've hopped down from her bed, marched over to Cheryl and inflicted injury, but it was lights out and she would've been caught. So instead she chewed on her fingers, muttering something about baby talking too much.

This sort of thing went on all the time with Cheryl and Denise. In a way, they were a welcome distraction from Dana, who was a bigmouth and thief. "She's *wicked*," I protested to my mother. But Dana was in the bed next to mine and my mother made me be nice to her. We were, as my mother put it, "stuck with each other." Problem was I could never spy her ripping me off. I knew she was a thief by the way she watched me. I didn't let on I was watching her watch, just went about my business, acting as if I didn't notice things missing — hard candy my grandmother bought at the Howard Johnson's. Some paper and pens. And money. Did she think I wouldn't notice?

Anyway, Dana got her period for the first time in the ward. There was a big fuss over it — curtains being pulled around her bed for privacy, nurses scurrying about, being nice to her. Not that it was unusual for the nurses to be nice. It's just that Dana was such a brat they usually had to yell at her.

There was talk about "her period."

"It's real heavy," one of them said.

"We'll have to change the sheets."

What could be so *heavy*, I wondered. And what in the world did any of this have to do with changing the sheets?

So the next day, when my mother came to visit, I asked. "Mom, what's a period?"

"Uh ..." she began, staring into the distance. "Well ... you sort of bleed."

Ah.

Mom didn't volunteer more information; I didn't ask. The obvious questions — where do you bleed *from*? and *why*? — went unanswered for a few more months. Until it started. In the cast.

Poor Gramma. She just happened to be babysitting at the time.

It was the look on her face, like she'd just discovered something rotted right there in the bed with me. What could be so horrid? I wondered. Had some creature quietly entered my room by night only to die and decay right there between my legs?

"You got your *menses*," my grandmother reported.

Menses? That was a new one on me. From the speed with which my grandmother turned and left, it was clear that It — whatever It was — would have to be removed immediately. Were supplies needed? Maybe a shovel to remove the carcass.

Instead my grandmother returned with the wash basin filled with steamy water, a washcloth and towels. I reached behind me for the prisms and the mirror and I watched.

My grandmother looked at me strangely, then dipped the cloth in the steamy soapy water. She wrung it, then started wiping as she did during a sponge bath. Did I pee all over myself? I wondered. But my grandmother wouldn't be grossed out by that. No, not the woman whose primary

concern was the consistency and quantity of bowel movements. My grandmother looked, twisted her neck, then
looked away.

As she dipped the cloth into the water, I caught a
glimpse of the bright red on the washcloth. But my grandmother continued, systematically wiping-dipping-wringing,
wiping-dipping-wringing.

Surely the sudden appearance of bright red blood was
significant, yet my grandmother showed no signs of concern.
Grimaces of disgust maybe, but not concern.

When she was through and had left the room, I removed
the glasses and held up the mirror to look at my face.

Zits. Still gross.

I put the prisms back on, then lowered the mirror to see
where all the red was coming from. *Exactly* where it was
coming from.

My right hand hovered a few moments before my fingers
crept inside my thigh and into my pubic hair. I found myself
scratching myself, sometimes where it itched, sometimes
where it didn't, my index and middle fingers separating into
a "V" over the softer parts, pressing more firmly and pulling
together, then clawing inward, toward that warm, full-feeling
place that wanted to be found.

Then my middle finger slipped inside my vagina.

I liked the feeling and kept it in, wiggled it around, then
wondered what would happen if my grandmother walked in.

I pulled out the finger and looked at it.

Bloody.

I brought it to my nose and smelled it. It was a strange odour, strong but not unpleasant and I had the feeling I was the only person who would think so. I smeared the finger on the sheet then examined the nail. There was a dark outline of blood around the cuticle.

I knew there would be no discussion about it. My grandmother just had one of those faces.

If it hadn't been for the look on my grandmother's face, I probably wouldn't have known my period started. So I asked my mother why she didn't tell me more about menstruation when I asked.

"I didn't think you'd start so soon."

"Why?"

"Well, you had so many other physical problems that I thought it would be different for you."

I thought that was strange, because except for the zits, I never really felt all that different.

Do I Smell?

Menstrual blood doesn't smell until it is exposed to air. Even then, the scent is not strong unless you go unwashed for a couple of days or leave your bloody pads sitting in an open garbage for a week! Because we have so many folds and crevasses in our vulvas, be sure to wash carefully. Take the time to enjoy a nice, long bath.

Some dogs notice the smell of menstrual blood and will go nosing about in open bathroom garbage pails if they smell a used pad or tampon. Yeesh! If you have a nosey pooch, make sure you have a bathroom garbage with a secure lid.

There are menstrual products with perfumes. However, these perfumes may cause irritations and allergic reactions in your tender vulva. Some women choose to use douches after they menstruate. A douche consists of a bag of scented liquid and a tube that is stuck up the vagina. The liquid is squeezed through the tube into the vagina. People believe that this washes the uterus and vagina, but actually infections have been linked to douche use. Douching is *completely unnecessary* because our vaginas clean themselves and douching will interfere with this natural process. Douching will not act as a birth control method either.

Each woman has her own natural scent depending on her body chemistry, mood and diet. It's okay to like your body odour!

A FUNNY FEELING

MANJIT KAUR

*Manjit Kaur was raised in Malaysia and now lives
in the United States with her husband. This is a
story about a Punjabi girl and her family. Jassy is feeling
confused about what's happening to her body. First there
is the funny feeling she gets around her handsome
neighbour. Then she gets a crampy feeling in her
stomach. People around Jassy are acting strangely too,
and she begins to wonder if there are
answers to all of these mysteries.
Certainly some of the stories Jassy has heard about
menstruation don't provide the right answers. You
cannot get pregnant from a boy if he touches you when
you're menstruating. And men cannot tell that a
woman is menstruating by her odour.*

MOHAN DAS STOOD on the verandah, practising his shots
against the wall of my parents' bedroom. He rolled the white
ball back and forth with his hockey stick, never getting tired

of the monotonous *tuk, tuk* rhythm. I liked the sound of the
ball hitting the white wall and then lightly tapping the solid
golden-brown hockey stick that gleamed from the coconut
oil Mohan Das must have rubbed into it. I looked at the
white wall my mother had recently painted, expecting to
find a bruise or deformation on it, but it seemed to be handling the assault fairly well.

I sat on the verandah of the two-bedroom house my parents rented and watched Mohan Das as I wove a rug for my
mother. It was almost five in the evening, the heat of the day
slowly lifting. For months now, I had been trying to put a
rug together for my mother, something similar to the beautiful one I had seen done by a Home Economics student at
the yearly school exhibition.

I sat on the cool cement with a gunny sack sprawled out
in front of me. My plastic bag filled with colourful remnants
of material sat right next to me. This had become my daily
routine: sitting outside watching the brilliant red sun fade
into the horizon and enjoying the sound from the ball while
I wove.

I looked up from cutting the remnants into two-by-four
strips when my mother came out of the house. She had a
hot steamy glass of tea in her hand. My mother lived on hot
tea with lots of milk and sugar in it. She bent at her waist
and placed the glass down on the floor. She then proceeded
to slowly lower herself onto the floor, careful not to aggra-
vate her weak knees. Her doctor had repeatedly told her
that she needed to lose some weight. Her knees were no

longer capable of handling her pear-shaped body, but the warning had not encouraged her to give up her indulgence in sugar.

"So, when are you ever going to get that rug done, Jassy?" My mother called me Jassy, short for Jasvinder. "I am tired of sticking your father's old T-shirts in front of the bathroom door."

"I'll get it done; I am almost half-way down the sack," I replied, pointing to the neat rows of colourful material I had sewn into the sack.

"Oh, it is just like you to do something half-way and then leave it. You never ever finish what you start. See what happened to the basket you were trying to make? It is lying in the cupboard half done. Typical of you! Always so eager to start something then you drop it half-way through."

I ignored my mother, embarrassed, wondering if Mohan Das had heard her. I was sure he had heard her, but was pretending that we were not even there. He kept on hitting the ball.

We sat there quietly, my mother slowly sipping her tea as she watched me thread my seven-inch needle with a strip of material. I struggled to get the strip of cloth through the rusty eye, my hands shaking violently because my mother sat next to me, watching me like a hawk. When I finally got the strip through, I tugged it further down so it would not slip out of the hole. Just then I experienced an odd sensation in my abdomen. I ignored the feeling. I looked up to find Mohan Das looking directly at me.

Mohan Das had never talked or looked at me before. I was startled to find him staring at me. I assumed he never paid much attention to me because I was only eleven years old. I found myself unable to hold his gaze so I looked down at my bag instead, shoving my hand into it pretending to find a piece that would match the strip I had just sewn.

"How is it coming along?" he asked, as he squatted in front of me.

I glanced sideways to see how my mother would react to him starting a conversation with me. I think part of the reason she did not mind having him around was that he usually left us alone while he waited for my father. I got really nervous when I noticed that my mother was not paying any attention to us. Where is my dad, I wondered. He was usually home by now so he and Mohan Das could go play a game of field hockey at the *padang* before it got dark. Mohan Das got rides to the hockey field from Dad who was always eager to give anybody a ride as long as they enjoyed playing hockey and took it seriously. Mohan Das was an avid hockey player. Without fail, rain or shine, he was bound to be at our door step in his bleached white shorts with his gleaming hockey stick at a quarter-to. This had been going on for months now and he had never talked to me before or showed any indication that he even knew I existed.

"Umm ... it is a little slow but I am almost done," I said bashfully. Mohan Das fingered the rug and I found myself staring at his brown hand, the hand that gripped the hockey stick so skilfully. He has strong hands, I thought, almost the same brown shade as the hockey stick. His fingers were long and slim, lined with little curly black hairs. My eyes traveled upwards from his hand to his arm, all the way to his face and I found myself staring into his dancing light brown eyes. All of a sudden I felt shyness creep up my spine so I shifted my eyes. My gaze fell onto his lips. His upper lip was thinner than the lower and I discovered that I instinctively wanted to reach out to touch them and feel their softness. Afraid that I would reach out unconsciously, I turned my gaze again. This time it fell on the cleft in his chin. Mohan Das was clean shaven, his five o'clock shadow barely visible. He was so close that I could faintly smell his aftershave cologne. I wondered what it was. Old Spice? Four Seven Eleven? My spine began to tingle and I felt goosebumps running up my back. What was happening to me? I had never felt this way before, especially towards Mohan Das.

At that moment, the odd sensation in my abdomen reappeared. I did not understand why I was getting this feeling. Something did not feel right. Maybe I am going to be sick, I thought. Then I felt a wetness in my pants. I wondered if I had wet my pants due to my nervousness of having Mohan Das so close to me. This was the first time I had ever had any man so close to me and I was nervous, but not enough to wet my pants. Something else is going on here, I thought. I had better go check. I slowly put the rug down on the floor and stood up. Mohan Das stood up too. I found it difficult to look up into his eyes, so with my heart in my throat I mumbled, "I need to get a drink of water."

I quickly went to the bathroom, undid my navy shorts and pulled my underwear down. I stood there for a few minutes unable to move, staring at the red stain on my underwear not sure what to do next. I had heard of menstruation; my friends and I had talked about it at school. The ones who were more physically mature became our teachers, educating us about the monthly goings-on in a woman's body. Well, this can't be my period, I thought. I am too young for it. Anyway, what does it even look like? I must have hurt myself or why else am I bleeding? I pulled on my clothes and went outside in search of my mother. She would know what to do.

"Ma, can you come in here for a while?" I asked her while I stood at the doorstep. I did not dare go outside for fear everyone would know what was going on. My best friend, Wilma, had said that men could smell the blood and I did not want Mohan Das to smell it.

"You come here," replied my mother.

"Ma, Auntie Rani needs you in here. She wants you to try on that new dress that she is making for you," I lied. Auntie Rani, my mother's younger sister, was making a dress for my mother, but she was far from having it done.

"Really, your Auntie Rani is getting so good at this. Why can't I have children like her? She is so good at everything she does and she always finishes whatever she starts," grumbled my mother as she tried to raise herself up. I stood inside the doorway not volunteering a hand to my mother as she struggled to stand up. She would kill me when she found out that Auntie Rani did not need her to try out the dress yet.

Auntie Rani had come here three years ago to attend nursing school in the town we lived in. Even though she lived in the hostel, she constantly visited us during her days off to sew Mother a dress or bake us something. My mother loved Auntie Rani because she was always doing something — baking, cooking, cleaning or studying. She felt that her children did not do as much as Auntie Rani did and since Auntie Rani was only eight years older than me, my mother treated her like her own child. Of course, I resented the constant comparison I had to face from my mother, that Auntie Rani was so good at this, so good at that and I, on the other hand, could never do anything right.

The minute my mother walked in the door I tugged her arm. "Ma," I stammered, not sure how to tell her what was going on. My mother loved jumping to conclusions so I had to be tactful or I could find myself in a lot of trouble. "Something is not right," I continued. "There is blood on my panties. I don't know how it got there." I quickly added as a defence, "I did not do anything, Ma."

My mother's eyes narrowed to a slit as she watched me for a few moments, not saying anything. Then she walked into the room where Auntie Rani was sitting slouched over the sewing machine. I was afraid so I did not follow her. Since she had not said a word, I did not know what she would do next. I definitely did not want to be near her just in case she swung her heavy arm around. My mother did not have much patience and constantly used her hand on us when she was in a bad mood. She whispered to Auntie Rani so I could not hear what she was saying.

Next thing I knew, both women were heading towards me. I cringed, waiting for some form of punishment to land on me, but my mother just walked past me. My aunt took my hand and led me to my bedroom. She told me to take my shorts off while she rummaged through her overnight bag. She pulled out a sanitary pad and showed me how to use it. We did not talk much. I was upset that my mother got her sister to show me what to do. I did not understand why my mother left me after I told her what had happened. Well, there really is not much to say, I thought as Auntie Rani showed me how to use the strap that held the pad in place.

"There you go, Jassy," said Auntie Rani when I was all dressed again. "You just had your first period and in a few hours you will need to change that pad. I would give you another pad, but that is the last one I have. You better go to the store soon before it gets dark," she said as she proceeded to leave.

"Can't I just use my mother's? I am sure she has them," I asked, trying to avoid going to the store. Sometimes my mother would send me to the store to get her some and I hated the way the guy at the store would wrap the sanitary box in old used newspaper before he handed it to me. He wrapped it so I would not be embarrassed carrying it home, but it only made things worse. As if the whole world could not guess what was rectangular and wrapped in newspaper...

"Your mother no longer has her period," she said and went back to the next room to resume her sewing.

I stood there glued to the floor, shocked. Slowly I began to understand why my mother did not want to have anything to do with me. It was not me, it was the menstruation. Come to think of it, in the last few months she had not sent me to the store to get her any pads. Finally things fell into place and I felt much better.

I walked to the cupboard in my room and stood facing the full length mirror on the front of the cupboard. My shorts felt stuffed as if I had something in there. Well, I *did* have something in there! I looked into the mirror to see if people would notice that I had my pad on. My dark shorts looked normal. I was glad I had navy blue shorts on. I couldn't wait to go to school tomorrow to tell all my friends about it.

Then I began to wonder if I should. My mother and aunt did not react as if they were thrilled about it; maybe I should not be thrilled either. All the horrible stories my friends talked about in class came back to me. When you started bleeding you had to be extra careful with boys. If you happened to sit next to one when you were menstruating and accidentally touched him you could get pregnant. Maybe that was why my mother wasn't too thrilled about it. Well, I had better get back to my rug.

I wasn't sure how to react when I got outside. I wondered if Mohan Das knew what was going on. I did not dare look into his face and he had resumed practising with the ball. My mother sat there calmly as if nothing had happened.

☉ The Arrival ☉

Just as I lowered myself down I heard that familiar honking
of my father's old yellow Peugeot. My father usually honked
a few doors away to let us know that he was almost home.

"The *Maharajah* is home. I don't understand why your
father needs to announce to the entire neighbourhood that
he is home," said my mother. "I am going to ask your dad to
stop by the market on his way home from hockey and pick
up some chicken. Tomorrow I will make you some chicken
soup. You will need it for strength," she added and placed
her chubby hand softly on my head.

My father pulled the car into the driveway, parking a few
feet from us. As he stepped out of his car I wondered if my
mother would tell him that I had started menstruating or if
he would just smell me and know.

Do Men Have Cycles Too?

Men DO have cycles. Like women's menstrual cycles, men have cycles that are created by the production of hormones. The sex hormones estrogen, progesterone and testosterone are found in both women and men's bodies: however, women have much more estrogen and progesterone, while men have much more testosterone. Sex hormones move through the body in a particular pattern or cycle. However, while a woman's cycle happens over a month or so, a man's cycle happens every single day!

Many young women think that men don't have as many things about their bodies to worry about as women. That depends on your perspective. During puberty, it takes some time for a boy's body to get used to the new flow of hormones. Boys going through puberty may ejaculate (release sperm from their penis) when sleeping, which is called a *wet dream*. Some boys find this a very shameful experience, as if they wet the bed, but it is quite natural and a sign of maturing into manhood. Young men also experience sudden erections, where their penises stick straight out, and this may cause embarrassing moments. They often feel that they must shave their facial hair every day even if they don't need to, and many are very concerned about their penis size or their height or muscles. Puberty is a very confusing time for boys too!

JENNIFER'S BIRTHDAY

TAMARA STEINBORN

*In "Jennifer's Birthday," Tamara Steinborn tells the
story of two sisters. Jennifer is older than Azalea, but
she's different from other kids her age. Because it
sometimes takes Jennifer longer to understand things,
Azalea watches over her to make sure she's okay.
And this year on Jennifer's birthday, the girls have
something special to celebrate.*

MY FAMILY WAS FILLED with boys and our lives were cluttered
with baseball gloves, Nintendo games and sports on Sundays.
My mother and father prayed for their firstborn to be a girl.
Then they prayed for a little sister. Then they prayed for a
girl to round off the family. By their fourth child they had
given up prayer and left everything to fate. The next child
was Jennifer. My mother and my grandmother had wanted
to name her Juniper because of the Juniper bushes which
surrounded the house, but my father put his foot down —
this tribute to nature was too much for him. Unfortunately,

when I was born my mother got her way in honouring nature with my name: Azalea.

We were all told to be patient with Jennifer — she was just slow. She is taking the world at her own leisure, my dad would say. From very early on I decided to watch over Jennifer. We stuck together in a secret conspiracy, littering the household with as many girl things as we could. We did our best to keep the domestic cosmos well balanced.

On Jen's twelfth birthday, Mom and I took her shopping for some birthday clothes to the big new mall. Since we lived in a small town, a visit to the new mall was an adventure for us and we intended to make the most of our girls' day out.

I went into the change-room with Jennifer every time she tried on a dress. She wanted an adult dress to go with the old lipstick she had scavenged from Mom's cosmetic bag. Mom didn't know this and as a birthday favour to Jennifer I decided to keep this secret.

I was struggling with the neckline of a dress that was hunched around Jenny's neck when she let out a muffled wail.

"Hold on, dummy, I have to get the buttons undone before I can take it off."

She ignored me and began dancing around frantically.

"Hmff" was all I could hear as I struggled to yank the dress over her head. Finally, giving up, I left her dancing around as I went to find Mom.

Mom was talking with the saleswoman. Happy to hand over the reins of power, I immediately told her what was going on. Mom hurried off to the change-room. I followed, suddenly miserable in my failure and angry at this wrinkle in the day. I could feel my position as Mom's reliable right hand slipping.

In the change-room, Jen was bundled up in a confusion of clothing, flailing about like a dangerous weapon. I watched in awe as Mom immediately took charge of the situation without even gasping at the sight of my sister.

"Jennifer!" she barked.

My sister snapped to attention at the sound of Mom's voice. She had managed to twist the dress around her body and she looked as if she were suffocating. I felt sorry for her as she gurgled and protested underneath her trappings. My mother lost no time in unwinding her from the mess.

Suddenly Mom stepped back and looked at me in surprise. I had no idea what was going on, but was fairly confident that I had done nothing wrong.

"Azalea, open my purse and get the package of Kleenex out for me, please."

My mother's voice was kind and gently commanding. It was the voice she always used when Jen peed her pants. As I rummaged through the purse, I wondered if Jen had peed on the dress she had been trying on. I handed Mom the Kleenex and moved closer to examine the situation. Jen's lower half was exposed and I stared at the rust streaks along the insides of her thighs. Mom was licking Kleenex and trying to wipe as much of this stuff off as possible.

"Azalea, check the dress to see if there is any blood on it, please."

Mom's voice was still calm, and by now Jen had stopped

her wailing and was making low moaning noises. I wondered if she was in pain. I could hear Mom whispering softly and cooing into her ears. This took its effect; my sister calmed down to only the occasional sniff. By now, Mom had dressed her in her own clothing and was preoccupied with positioning the Kleenex in Jen's underwear. This act was of incredible interest to me and I observed my mother's movements with fascination. My sister snuffled, looked at me and suddenly burst out in laughter.

"Peed my pants and it stings!" she told me and chortled to herself.

I looked at my mother who looked at me and we both gave each other the "play along" signal. I handed the spotless dress back to Mom and she hung it neatly back on the hanger.

She had a look on her face that I will always remember. Taking Jen's hand and mine, we walked out together, my mother looking as if, after so many boys, she had finally had her motherhood justified. This is how I remember that look, how I have grown to understand that look.

ANEMIA

Anemia is a condition people get when they don't have enough of the mineral iron in their bodies. An anemic person feels very tired and looks pale, may have memory problems, dizziness and headaches, and may be short-tempered. Heavy menstruation or simply not getting enough iron in your diet can make you anemic.

To prevent anemia, eat plenty of foods that have iron, like lean meats (liver), leafy vegetable greens (spinach), whole-grain breads and dried fruit. Some women find that they need to take iron pills to prevent anemia. You can find iron pills at any drug or health-food store. If you already take a multi-vitamin, this probably has all the iron you need for a day. Check the label and be cautious about how much iron you take! Sometimes iron can make you constipated. Eat lots of fruit and drink lots of water to cure constipation.

REACHING OUT

*Having your period shouldn't be a lonely, scary experience.
When you get your first period, it's probably a good time to
share your feelings and learn some tips from people who
know what to do. Sisters and moms and best friends are
great people to talk with, but they aren't the only ones who
can help when you find yourself in an awkward situation.
And who knows — maybe some day you can help someone
else understand what having periods is all about.*

Outrunning Gravity

MARY HELEN STEFANIAK

*In "Outrunning Gravity," Mary Helen Stefaniak tells
the story of a father and daughter. Kelly's father is
feeling a bit lonely and confused as he watches her grow
up. Kelly's first period arrives while her mother is away.
When Kelly must turn to her dad for help, they both
learn that though she is no longer a child,
Kelly and her father can still be good friends.*

"LOOK, DAD, IT'S NOT THAT I don't want to go camping
with you."

Kelly put her fork down and stopped chewing long
enough to bite her lower lip and place her hand over mine on
the table. Her touch was a rare treat. In the month and a half
since her eleventh birthday — for which she had received
three sets of matching bras and panties — physical contact

between us had grown less frequent and more awkward every day. Last night when she kissed me good night, she missed my cheek completely in her haste and kissed the air beside my ear instead. Now she was patting my hand with what at least seemed to be affection.

"We've been planning this for months, Kelly," I said.

"I know, I *know*. But Mrs Burns said no weekend rehearsals until November. How was I supposed to know she'd change her mind this afternoon?" This was my pre-teenage daughter talking to her almost middle-aged father using the old victim-of-circumstance, my-hands-are-tied ploy. I'd used it often myself.

"But you've never been camping in the fall, Kelly. You don't know what you're missing. No bugs, crisp mornings, cool nights, leaves turning colour and everything. We'd have a great time." I meant to sound enticing but I seemed to be pleading. "Just you and me, kid."

"Dad," she said, looking me squarely in the eye as she sat facing the bay window, her eyes bluer than possible in the light. "I have a —" she hesitated, no doubt searching her mind for something Director Burns had said to cast and crew "— I have a *commitment* to the play." She sat up straighter, pleased with herself. "People are counting on me."

"I was counting on the weekend, Kelly."

She looked sadly at the remains of the taco dinner for a moment then flicked a shred of cheese across the table at me. "I've got it! Let's go camping *next* weekend. Mrs Burns is going to be out of town, she told us. Let's go then." She smiled and showed her mother's dimples. Her hair bounced around behind her plastic headband. "Just you and me, Dad."

"I'm sure your mother will go for that in a big way. She gets home on Wednesday and we take off Friday?" I was pouting outright now.

"We could all three of us go ...," she began. I didn't even bother to respond. She sighed pointedly — she learned that one from me, too — and pushed back her chair, making it squeal on the wooden floor.

I ate my last taco alone without worrying about whether I got sauce on my moustache. ("Ooh, Daddy, that's *gross*.") I was a little ashamed of myself, but I had been counting on the weekend for more than crisp mornings and autumn leaves. What else can you do to keep in touch with a daughter who's wearing matching bras and panties? I'd pictured us huddled close to a campfire, watching the stars, hiking the old Scuppernong Trail together, eating our biscuits and cheese beside the creek, scooping icy water from a spring that bubbled up through the sand.

Kelly poked her head through the doorway from the den as I was wiping my moustache. "Besides," she said, "it's supposed to rain all weekend. I heard it on the radio."

She kept trying to make it up to me. She cleared the table and washed the dishes while I brooded in a beanbag chair in front of *Hogan's Heroes*. She brought me a beer, already opened. Peace offerings, I thought, remembering candy bars and piggyback rides. Bribery. Appeasement. I barely grunted thanks. I didn't even yield later when, standing over a scoured sink and gazing out the window, I saw her outside in the dusk, cleaning the dog's pen. When she came back in and headed straight for the bathroom to wash her hands I hid out in the den with my beer and my reruns.

I watch a lot of TV lately, mostly old sitcoms. They don't make them like that any more. Good thing they don't, Kelly says. When she complains about my choice of programs I like to remind her that she used to watch *Hogan's Heroes* sitting on my lap while we waited for Mom to come home from school. Kelly wrinkles her nose at that and tells me that I'm living in the past. What's wrong with the past, I'd like to know. In the past I had a head full of hair and legs that could do a mile in 4.67 minutes. In the past she was an adorable (and adoring) toddler with curly pigtails — eleven year old Kelly groans at the thought and tugs a lock of her hair straight.

She stayed in the bathroom a long time, much longer than necessary to wash her hands, although I probably wouldn't have noticed if I hadn't come out to the kitchen for another beer and heard the banging and slamming coming from behind the bathroom door. After I popped the top off the can I waited for a minute by the refrigerator, listening. There weren't enough drawers and cabinets in there for her to be looking for something so long. The racket was finally reduced to one rhythmical banging of what sounded like the same door, over and over again. I put down my beer and walked down the hall.

"Kelly?"

There was no answer, but the banging stopped immediately. I waited another moment and tapped politely on the door.

"Kelly, are you all right?"

Long pause. Then, very quietly: "Yeah."

"What were you — I mean, were you opening and closing the cabinets in there for some reason?"

"Yes."

"Looking for something?"

"No."

"Kelly?"

No answer.

"Then what was all that banging?"

Still no answer.

"Kelly, what were you looking for?"

"Never mind."

I stood outside the door, listening for telltale sounds from the other side, wondering what she might have gotten herself into. (I remembered a haircut she'd given herself when she was five.) When she spoke up again in a small, quivering voice, I could barely make out the words.

"I want my mother," she said.

It was not what I expected to hear, under the circumstances. Not that Kelly doesn't love her mother, but the two of them have always had a stormy relationship, right from the beginning, when Anne had to juggle her studies around a toddler who found no one more interruptible than a mother hunched over a book. Kelly had learned early to run to me for solace or amusement: Dad the Entertainer, the living Diversionary Tactic. Lately though, she and Anne had taken to going shopping together or swimming at the Y. The other day I caught them giggling over a photograph album with my college track pictures and newspaper clippings in it.

"What's so funny?" I asked them.

They just looked at each other, then at me, and as if on cue, shook their heads and giggled some more. I didn't let on but they hurt my feelings.

Now, though, the quiver in my daughter's voice got to me. I leaned against the bathroom door.

"Kelly, what's the matter, honey? Can I help?"

"*No!*"

So much for tenderness. Now I was mad. "Kelly Anne, you stop this fooling around right now and come out of there!"

"I can't."

"Why not?"

She shouted, "Because I just got my period, that's why! — oh god." Her voice fell at the end.

I felt pretty dumb then, not so much for failing to guess the problem as for the little shock I felt when she told me what it was. My mind flashed back to fourth grade when they put all of us boys into one room and the girls into another and showed everybody one of those animated documentaries Walt Disney used to put out called "The Secret of Life" or "You're Growing Up Now!" The cartoon woman whose reproductive system got cross-sectioned and explained always looked alarmingly like Snow White. I remembered too how we fourth-graders squirmed on our metal chairs as we learned that it was nothing to be upset or embarrassed about, that it was a beautiful and natural thing.

I cleared my throat.

"Kelly, honey, is this your first —" I almost said *time* "— your first one? Period, I mean?"

"Yes. Oh, Daddy."

She was weeping. She'd been in the bathroom for half an hour now. Something I read once about women being prisoners of their own biology popped into my head.

"Well," I said. "All right." I thought a minute. "Doesn't your mother have something in there that you can use?"

I heard her weeping more loudly.

"I'm sure I saw a box under the sink."

"Not any more," she wailed. "I wrecked all of 'em."

"I don't understand," I said.

"I can't get them in!" she said, and burst into a new level of tears and sobbing.

I wished Anne were home. Then I said, "Kelly, you just sit tight. I'll be right back."

"Where are you going?" She sounded alarmed, as if I might be abandoning her to the bathroom, or worse, running next door to get Mrs Kaminski.

"I'm going to the store."

I am not the sort of man who feels embarrassed about buying feminine products if his wife puts them on the grocery list, but whisking down the aisle to pluck Anne's tampons off the shelf is an entirely different matter from lingering there to examine boxes of *mini* and *maxi pads*. I had to read the directions and recommended uses on the back of each package, checking out the actual-size pictures to see exactly what was inside. I think I was hoping for one marked "Beginners." A couple of women looked at me strangely as they reached past to grab their brand; I'd look up quickly to see what they had chosen.

In the end I bought them all: seven boxes of different brands and sizes, with pictures on the front of women riding bicycles or jogging — more Kelly's style, I thought, than the ones in billowy dresses floating through fields of flowers. I wanted to be sure I'd have the right thing for an eleven year old girl crying in the bathroom. The checkout clerk, a pregnant young woman, gave me a small smile as the bagger, a skinny teenage boy, divided my purchases into two light but bulky bags.

At home Kelly opened the bathroom door just wide enough to let me push the boxes through. She didn't comment on the number although she thought I was finished after the fifth one and started to close the door. When all seven were inside she said, "Thanks, Dad." I heard the lock click.

I stood there in the hallway for a moment not quite knowing what to do, not quite feeling like the rescuer I had thought myself to be. Then I went back to the kitchen to the refrigerator and took out the beer I'd started before I left for the store. I sat down at the table with my fingers growing numb around the cold can and found myself thinking sentimental thoughts like: Where has the time gone? And: My little Kelly is all grown up. But when I thought them, they weren't sentimental; there was a hardness in my throat, a sinking in my stomach. I thought about Kelly sitting on the floor in my workroom when she was two, showering herself with wood shavings while I built her a dollhouse she never played with. I thought about the small of her back on my palm in the pool. *Lay your head back, Kelly. Relax. Trust me.*

I remembered a camping trip when she was hardly more than a baby and I took her for a piggyback ride through the woods. When our path ended at a ravine, I hesitated for an instant at the edge, then said, "Hang on tight!" and plunged downward. It was much steeper than it looked from the top. The only way I could keep from falling was to try to outrun gravity, hooking one hand and then the other around passing tree trunks to break our speed, thinking all the while that if I tripped and fell, we'd roll and bounce the rest of the way down; if Kelly didn't let go, I'd crush her.

She didn't let go. All the way down she shrieked in my ear and clung so tightly to my neck that she choked me. When I landed on my hands and knees in the stream at the bottom, she rolled off my back into the water. I grabbed the front of her T-shirt and she came up sputtering and laughing, her pigtails like two dripping dog ears. She wanted to do it again.

"Daddy."

I turned around in my chair. She was standing in the doorway, looking shy and a little sheepish, but no more or less womanly than she had before. Her hands were jammed in the pockets of her jeans, her T-shirt was a little snug across her chest and her hair fell wild and curly almost to her shoulders, barely restrained by that purple plastic band. I wanted to ask her if she was all right and if I bought the right thing, but there seemed to be no right words to say it with. We looked at each other.

"So," I said finally. "Did you get everything squared away?"

My daughter laughed at me. Then she came around behind my chair and folded her arms around my neck. She hugged me so hard she choked me a little.

THE CHLORINE REPORT

Most tampon and pad makers bleach the cotton they use for their products with chlorine to make them whiter. This process is very bad for the environment. It's possible that chlorine and other chemicals found in pads and tampons might be bad for your sensitive vulva too, although we don't know for sure because good studies have not yet been done. You can find *unbleached* tampons and pads at health-food stores and some grocery stores.

CAN YOU REALLY FLUSH TAMPONS DOWN THE TOILET?

While most tampon manufacturers claim that you can, it depends on the plumbing. Some toilet pipes, particularly in old buildings, are narrower than others and tampons get stuck easily causing backups. Tampons are also bad news for septic tanks, so don't flush them if your home or cottage has septic plumbing. If you have doubts, wrap the used tampon in toilet paper and throw it in the garbage. Most public washrooms have a special litter bin for your menstrual pads and applicators, usually found right in the stall next to the toilet.

It's important to remember that *pads* and *plastic* tampon applicators cannot be flushed down the toilet. Pads plug up plumbing. (How embarrassing when the toilet overflows!!) Plastic tampon applicators look small and harmless but they can be very dangerous for wildlife. These applicators pass easily through sewage waste disposal systems and end up in our oceans and rivers where birds and animals mistake the plastic for food. Plastic cannot be digested and often hurts an animal's digestive system. Millions of birds and thousands of animals die each year from eating plastic.

A Passage to Womanhood

CHI NGUYEN

*Chi Nguyen, the author of this story, is sixteen years
old. In "A Passage to Womanhood," Chi remembers
what it was like when she got her first period.
At twelve, Chi feels that she has it made. Getting her
period makes her feel older and more mature, and Chi
wants to keep this special feeling all to herself. But then
her younger sister gets her period at eleven and their
mother leaves it to Chi to explain the details.*

PICTURE THIS. A week after my twelfth birthday, I got IT.
My sign of womanhood — my first period.

Up until then all I'd heard were tidbits, little rumours of
how my life was going to change. I was soooo excited. Chi
Nguyen is now a WOMAN, I thought. For the next couple of
weeks I ran around the house and stood taller, felt stronger

and appeared prouder. For once, I had something no one else could ever have.

Or not!

What I thought was my own special thing seemed to be happening to all of the girls in my class. One by one, we joined the sacredness of womanhood.

So, a new tradition had begun in my life. Ah, that wonderful cycle of menstruation. Just think, I told myself, every month I'll get to feel proud and special. Except for the mood swings. The cramps. And the backaches.

Reality began to sink in.

Well, I thought, at least I've got something to hold over my sister's head.

I have always felt some jealousy towards my sister Diane. She is an extremely quiet, shy and reserved girl. She's more respected by our parents because she is more passive than I am. She can keep her lips shut. She's more focussed in school. She gets along better with my brother. Oh, and of course, when we were younger Diane had all of the Barbie dolls. The only advantage I have ever had over her is that I will always be the oldest and therefore, know so much more about life than she will.

The years passed by and my little sister got her first period. It was three months after her ELEVENTH birthday! Eleven years old? I was twelve when I got mine. This isn't fair, I thought. How come she's a woman before me?

Diane was sitting on the toilet, a little dazed. My mother was with her and was confused too. She was shocked to realize that her little girl had grown up.

Mom called me into the bathroom and simply said, "Take care of her. Show her what to do."

At first I laughed but it was a nervous giggle. Then I became annoyed. Just when I had become accustomed to the higher status of womanhood, my sister had to go and get her period. But the more I thought about it, the more it became clear to me. Diane was a WOMAN now. And she was in need of my help!

I wasn't really sure what to do. What was I to say that she wouldn't already know? She had puberty classes in school, television, books and workshops.

So I decided to show her all of the tips that I had learned from my MANY years of experience. Yes, anything over two years constitutes a wealth of knowledge!

"There's, um, pads... here take these. You'll probably find these most comfortable." I handed her a pad. "You stick it to your underwear." She gave me a doubtful look.

"I'm serious. Their whole purpose is to soak up whatever comes out." She was not impressed.

"And your other options are these," I said as I held up a box of tampons. "You basically shove these up inside you. Don't worry, they can be awkward at first and they take some getting used to. Stick with the pads until you're more comfortable."

I couldn't tell how she was taking all of this. She seemed completely unfazed by the whole incident.

"Well," I said. "You've joined the ranks. You're now a woman. Congrats."

All I could do was hope that my speech was good enough. Getting your period is a life-changing occurrence and it's not something you should have to go through alone. So I added, "If you need anything, *just ask,* okay?" She was still my little sister after all.

Then we had a pillow fight and, of course, being the oldest, I whipped her to shreds and declared myself winner. Maybe — if she's lucky — someday I'll share with her the secrets of pillow fighting too.

TAMPON USERS BE AWARE

Tampons are convenient and some women just love them. However, there are health risks involved. If you use tampons or are thinking about it, here's some important stuff you should know.

- Some plastic applicators have been known to pinch or cut the inside of the vagina. Paper applicators won't do this although they may not be as easy to insert.
- Tampons that are too absorbent scrape your vagina when you pull them out and can damage your

(cont'd)

vagina, or they may absorb all your vagina's moisture and cause sores. You can tell a tampon is too absorbent if it's hard to pull out, if it comes apart when you remove it, or if your vagina feels dry and sore. To avoid this, use the lightest absorbency you can, change your tampon brand, vary tampon use with pad use, or stop using tampons altogether.

- **Toxic Shock Syndrome** (TSS) is a rare but very dangerous illness. It's thought to be caused by a bacteria that infects the vagina. Most cases of TSS have been associated with tampon use. The material used in some tampons, especially the high absorbency kind, are just the sort of home this deadly bacteria likes.

The symptoms of TSS are high fever, vomiting, diarrhea, sudden low blood pressure and a peeling, sunburn-like rash. Women have died from TSS. Teenage girls have the highest risk of getting TSS because your young bodies can't fight the bacteria as well as fully matured women's bodies can.

But, *you can protect yourself:* change your tampon every four hours or less, use a tampon with a light absorbency, and use pads when you can.

THE SPAGHETTI TEST

COLETTE HARRIS

*Colette Harris' short story, "The Spaghetti Test," is set in
England, her birthplace. In the story, Helen is teased by
other students because she seems different and awkward.
And when she gets her first period, Helen is terrified.
Fortunately, help arrives just in time.
A note: in England, sanitary pads are
called "towels"; sweaters are called "jumpers";
and underpants are called "knickers."*

SHE LOOKED WEIRDER that day than I'd ever seen her. In the
saline humidity of a school change-room in summer, here
was Spag without her spagginess. For once she wasn't slim-
ing. She was scared witless.

She was a lonely girl who always seemed to be ever
pudgy, ever baby-like, tottering from person to hostile person

like a toddler that loses its Mum in a department store. That's why someone had one day called her "The Spaghetti Test": the harder you threw her against the wall of unfriendliness, the more grimly she'd stick. And unfortunately for her, so did the name. It made her a kind of legend and it stopped classmates from taking her seriously.

I just got used to finding her faintly repulsive. I think it was the sense of huge effort she exuded and the way her Boris Becker blond eyelashes made her sausage-skin face look permanently surprised. The way she boggled and bulged when she spat down the school trumpet, only to sit down beaming with pleasure after a wobbly solo said it all. She was somehow too old as well as too young to fit in with the rest of the message-swapping sex detectives amongst her fourteen year old peers.

That day in the change-room, after a particularly horrific fifteen hundred metres on the wilting playing field, she told me she was dying. And I almost laughed. Visions of her puffing chubby effort in sports lessons loomed before my eyes. Her corned-beef legs in the whipping winter wind of a netball lesson. The sideways tilt of her head; so grateful when she got picked for a team before she was the last one on the sidelines.

But then I saw the way she was goose-pimpled even in the sultry clogginess of the locker room and my eyes travelled down to where she was clutching at the crotch of her athletic shorts. It hit me then that this wasn't funny.

"I'm dying," she said. "There's blood down there and it's

all unhealthy, not red, and I've got a backache and my belly
hurts ...." She trailed off into dry raspings that hiccupped
out of her. Comparisons with spaghetti became irrelevant as
I looked at her suddenly tragic face. My God, I thought, she
doesn't know about periods.

How was I going to explain to her that her starchly crisp
mother had left her wide open for this kind of shock? I
wanted to scream at the woman who had forced Helen to do
chores and music practice from five until eight in the morning so she'd never be the sort to find teen mags exciting. For
her there had been no consumer surveys of tampons and
towels or the glimmering adverts about how all-day freshness
gives you the confidence to be your own woman.

I thought with relief and a ripple of love about the way
my mum had often embarrassed me by putting billowing
towels into overnight bags when I went to stay with friends.
I thought that no one in the street could possibly fail to
know that they were lurking in there. Her reply to my flam-
ing cheeks had been an earnest, "You never *know*, do you?"

And on the plane home from a school skiing holiday a
few weeks before this change-room bombshell, I had been
giddily proud when I realized that the nausea I had been suf-
fering from was directly related to the fact that I'd *started.*

Even someone as clued up as me had taken a while to
fathom it out though. I had thought for a while that I'd suddenly become incapable of wiping my arse properly and that
these were humungous skid marks. I made an effort to
record the times when I had only pissed so I'd know that any

brownish patches on my pants weren't signs of a mysterious sphincter disability or the remarkably shiny toilet paper. The difference between my confusion and Spag's total fear lay in the fact that I was hardly daring to hope that it might at last have happened, that I might be a real *woman* instead of just a girl!

Now I could sweep out of classrooms with an obvious bulge in my jumper sleeve, like Sarah Everton, and let the rest of them know that I'd *arrived*. The dreams of adulthood that had surfaced when I first found a silvery trail in the cotton of my Holly Hobby knickers had finally come true.

And Mum flew down the stairs shouting, "Well done!" when I announced it. I wondered what the reptile mother would say to this young woman and thought about what she should already have said.

So in the clinging musk of that change-room I said, "Don't cry, Helen," and put my arm around her. "It's only natural and it happened to me not long ago. It's called your 'period' or 'that time of the month' and stuff. It's nothing nasty. It just means that we're growing up. Do you want one of my sanitary towels?"

She said, "Yes please." And then she asked me what they were for.

Alternative Menstrual Moments:

Less than a century ago, pads were home-made from cloth and attached to the underwear with safety pins or tied to a cloth belt. Bloodstained pads were soaked in cold water, hand washed and hung to dry. This way, the cloth pads could be reused for each period. Your grandmother likely used cloth pads for her periods when she was a young girl.

Then came the "throw-away" pad. This was something that had to be bought at drugstores or pharmacies, and in the early days, was stored behind the counter (like prescription pills today!). There were no fancy adhesive strips (the sticky stuff that attaches the pad to your underwear) on the earliest disposable pads. Instead, women had to buy a special elastic belt that went around the waist and had attachments at either end to hold the pad in place. Your mother and your aunts likely used an elastic belt and pad when they were younger.

Today we have a huge assortment of store-bought pads and tampons that we can choose from. But history has come full circle. Now, some women aren't happy with the menstrual products that are available at the drugstore. They're concerned for the environment, for their health and for their wallets! Here are some alternatives to typical store-bought pads and tampons.

(cont'd)

- Your grandmother will think you're crazy, but cloth pads are back in style! They're so cheap compared to store-bought paper pads and they're *much* better for the environment. You can find them at health-food or environmental stores. Or you can make your own pads with terry cloth towels or the absorbent cotton fabric used for diapers. Use Velcro fasteners or pin the pad to your undies. When you remove it, soak the pad in cold water, then put it in the washing machine with your other clothes for a final wash. Like regular pads, cloth pads should be changed frequently. Keep a special bag in your purse or backpack to hold a spare pad and the used pad if you are changing it away from home. Cloth pads are ideal for those who don't have a heavy menstrual flow. If you have a heavy flow, a cloth pad may be used with a tampon.

- The Keeper: Another alternative method is called The Keeper. This is a small cup made of soft rubber that is inserted like a tampon into the lower part of your vagina to collect your menstrual blood. The cup should be emptied regularly and cleaned in warm water. Go to your local health-food store for details.

THE CHALLENGE

Having your period can sometimes be a real challenge.
It may demand fast thinking when it comes as a surprise.
Or it can require deep thinking when you uncover
some of the silly ideas people have about bleeding.
Getting your period can also give you the boost that
you need to get beyond the other challenges that
life can dish up. The stories in this section are about
young women who discover their own strengths and
convictions when they get their first periods.

On My Own

KARYN SILZER

*Karyn Silzer is a high school student. In "On My Own,"
she tells the story of how, a few years ago when she was
thirteen, she discovered that periods don't always come
when you want them to. Just when she is busiest, Karyn
finds that she's begun menstruating for the first time. It's
enough to make a girl crazy! But in having to deal with
this situation, Karyn also discovers that she's a lot more
resourceful and independent than she's ever dreamt.*

IT WAS A NORMAL SCHOOL day in late October of my grade
eight year.

Just like every other school day, the bell rang at 8:30. We
students had ten minutes to get to homeroom before the second bell at 8:40, followed by the announcements.

When the first bell rang on this particular day I was in
the office joking around with my friend, Suzanne. She and I
were responsible for reading the announcements over the PA
system to the entire school every other morning. We were

specifically chosen out of our entire grade for this duty and it was an honour and a big responsibility, although it also meant no more sleeping in.

As we were getting prepared that day I suddenly got a sharp pain in my stomach — well, at least I *thought* it was my stomach — but I ignored it because I had my mission: the announcements. Over the PA I told people to begin to proceed to their homeroom for the national anthem.

I tried to ignore my stomach but it hurt again and it was getting worse. When I finished with the announcement, I decided to go to the bathroom. Maybe this will make my stomachache go away, I thought. I had about ten minutes to spare. I told Suzanne where I was going and that I'd be back soon.

I went to the girls' bathroom across the hall from the office and entered one of the stalls. As I sat down I realized that I wasn't feeling particularly well. Then when I wiped I saw the blood!

Although my mom had told me that I would be starting my period soon this was definitely a *big* surprise. At thirteen it was about time. I was one of the last of my friends to start. In the previous months I thought I had started menstruating but I only had cramps, nothing else. While I wasn't looking forward to the rest of my life spent menstruating, I still wanted to get my period. Especially since all of my friends had it. But *now*?! What awful timing. As I sat there the only thing I could think was: "Why now when I only have a few minutes to get back to the announcements?"

For a moment I was really upset. I wanted someone to help me. I felt that I didn't know what to do. I wanted to cry.

But then I reminded myself that I had to be back in the office to do the announcements in about seven minutes. "Maybe I can handle this on my own," I thought. I pulled myself together. I had to! I had a time line to meet!

Fortunately, since my mom told me I would be getting my period soon, I — always cautious — had started carrying a pad in my backpack. Now I had to go to my locker where my backpack was to get the pad. But my locker seemed so far away: all the way upstairs and down two hallways. I never thought I could get there and back in only seven minutes. What was I going to do?

I'm wasting time thinking, I decided. And time is exactly what I can't afford to waste!

I started the trek to my locker. I was so afraid that I was going to leak through my pants that I waddled. Somehow I thought that holding my thighs together when I walked would slow the blood flow. I know now that I didn't need to worry about leaking because there really wasn't a lot of blood, but how was I supposed to know that then? Even if waddling wasn't necessary, it made me feel like I was doing *something* to help combat the situation.

I waddled upstairs and then as I waddled down the hall, I was greeted by my friends on their way to homeroom. I could have sworn they all knew my situation and were going to laugh — at least at the way I was walking — but no one seemed to notice.

☻ The Challenge ☻

Finally I got to my locker. It had only taken me about a minute, but it felt like an *eternity*. The clock was ticking! I tried to open the lock, but due to the Other Thing on my mind I forgot my combo. Finally I got the lock undone and opened the door. I turned to see if anyone was looking — left, right. When I was sure no one was near, I turned myself sideways. With my hip almost halfway into my locker, I fiddled to get my backpack open and, grabbing the pad, I shoved it into my pants pocket. Mission (almost!) accomplished. And without a single witness.

Then, just as I was about to leave, two of my friends from homeroom came up behind me. They asked me why I wasn't in the office getting ready to do the announcements. This is not the time to chat! I thought. I have a job to do! While trying to remain calm and in control I told them that I had forgotten something in my locker and had come up to get it. They wanted to talk, but I told them I was in a hurry.

As they left, I went to shut my locker. It was then that I noticed that they had closed the lock on the hook. Nice friends! Usually I'd find this humorous, but not today, *not now*. I had to open the lock again before I could close the locker. Talk about stress! I had a time line, and time was running out. I had to *be* somewhere!

Another eternity later, I got the lock open and shut the door, snapped the lock on and began to waddle back down to the washroom. When I finally got there a little bit of relief came, but not much. I was still running against the clock and my heart was pounding.

I ran into the stall and pulled the pad out from my pocket. It took me a second to figure it out, but it was pretty self-explanatory. Then I pulled on my pants and discovered that the pad was really uncomfortable. So bulky! I felt like I was walking funny (again!). I was certain that everyone would know something was up. I didn't want to go out into the halls. I felt like I was the only one who had ever had to deal with this. I felt so alone!

Then I heard the second bell ring and Suzanne say on the PA, "Please stand for the national anthem."

My time was up! The announcements were waiting! I calmed down and stopped myself from crying even though I wanted to. I washed my hands and bolted out of the washroom, across the hall and back into the office.

Reading the announcements — a task that should only take a few minutes — seemed to take a life time. Usually calm and focussed, I couldn't concentrate. My mind was all over the place. I couldn't keep a thought in my head long enough to remember it.

But then as I was saying "This concludes your morning announcements" I realized that I had made it! I had managed it all — the period, the pad, the announcements — and all on my own! I still wanted to cry and I wanted to tell someone. But now I knew I could handle it.

When I left the office I took a drink from the fountain and said goodbye to Suzanne in the hall. She smiled and waved as if nothing at all had happened. She hadn't noticed! Somehow I had handled all this and no one knew anything was different. "Now *that*," I thought, "is a mission well accomplished." I smiled and, *this time*, I walked confidently down the hall to my first class, stopping now and then to chat and laugh with friends.

MENSTRUAL MYTH #1

False: You can't swim when you have your period.
Fact: You can swim, play basketball, do karate or anything you want when you have your period. When swimming, try using a tampon. Pads absorb water just as well as they absorb blood, so don't wear a pad in the pool!

MENSTRUAL MYTH #2

False: You can't have sex when you've got your period.
Fact: Women can have sex when they have their periods. Some women choose not to for various personal reasons while others really enjoy sex when they're bleeding. Remember: having sex is a choice you make and it's a choice that requires some careful thinking and preparation. Remember also always to protect yourself from unwanted pregnancy and sexually transmitted diseases.

MENSTRUAL MYTH #3

False: Cramps are all in your head.

Fact: Anybody who has ever had them can assure you that cramps are real. And there are a lot of women out there who have them regularly. Cramps aren't located in your head; rather you can find them under your belly button, near your hip bones!

Doctors think menstrual cramps may be caused by too much of a body chemical called prostaglandin. Prostaglandin may cause the uterus to contract painfully, cutting off oxygen to the muscles. However, other studies show that women in North America and Western Europe get cramps more than any other women in the world or in history, so cramps could be related to high fat diets and little exercise. But no one really knows for sure what causes cramps. More research needs to be done.

THE CURSE

MARY ALICE WARD

*Sometimes other people would like us to believe
that menstruation is dirty or shameful. People may be
obvious about their disgust, or their attitude may be
shown in little ways we hardly notice. Sometimes
places or people we greatly respect treat menstruation
as if it were dirty or abnormal. Even as a young
woman, Mary Alice Ward knew that this attitude was
wrong. In her story, Mary Alice describes the experiences
that she had with her first periods and how she found
ways to show those around her that menstruation was
not something bad, but powerful and special.*

I WAS A THIRTEEN YEAR OLD seventh-grader at West Junior
High School. What I knew about periods was limited to the
pamphlets distributed by the Kotex company. Every girl in
the Mesa county school district received such a pamphlet in
May of the sixth grade. The pamphlet described the biological process that occurred during menstruation and reassured

me that their product was the best defence against such a messy process. The pamphlet did not deal with what my biological process meant, at least not overtly. The pamphlet did not mention that I could now become a mother nor did it welcome me to the sisterhood of women. However, the pamphlet did have a covert message; using words like "protection," "security" and "sanitary," it communicated the notion that menstruation was an invasion of some sort and a dirty one at that. After reading the pamphlet, I had a vague idea that something called my "uterus" was one day going to "slough off" and I needed to protect myself against it.

You'd think I'd have known more about the subject given that I had an older sister and a mother who was a nurse. In our case, however, culture took precedence over medical training. My mother raised us the Armenian way, just as she had been raised. She didn't discuss menstruation until you began menstruating. At this point you joined the ranks of the "cursed" and could commiserate about it. With this limited information, I found myself in the pink bathroom after school with my sister talking about boys and going to the bathroom. It was my sister who noticed my stained underwear.

"Gross!" she sneered.

"Leave me alone," I snarled back, embarrassed. "I couldn't help it! I must have the flu." I had noticed a vague stomach-ache that day and had thought the stains must have been an "accident."

"You don't have the flu," Karen laughed. "You have the *curse*! You know — your period, Stupid!"

☙ The Challenge ☙

My embarrassment over having an "accident" was replaced with humiliation that I was too stupid even to know when I had gotten my own period. Tears sprang into my eyes.

Seeing my distress my sister said, "It's not a big deal, Mimi, mellow out. Here's what you do." She then proceeded, in a big-sisterly way, to instruct me in the use of the dreaded belt and Kotex. My "protection" was incredibly uncomfortable and bulky, like wearing a diaper. Shame burned my cheeks. I was certain everyone would be able to see that I had my period. My sister then showed me the best way to get blood off your underwear — cold water and soap scrubbed with a nail brush.

"And don't leave your underwear hanging on the rod because if Dad sees it he gets mad, so hang it on a hanger in your closet."

I was starting to get angry about this whole thing. The smouldering shame of a few moments earlier was developing into the slow burn of frustrated anger. With hot tears stinging my eyes I retreated to my room, turned on my radio and sulked.

I could hear my sister clambering down the stairs shouting, "Mo-o-om, Mimi's got the *curse*!"

Her voice made me shudder, but I was glad she was telling my mother. I expected my mom to drop whatever she was doing and come to my rescue, like she did when one of us was throwing up. I wanted her to come hold my head with one cold hand on my forehead and the other cold hand on the back of my neck. I felt like throwing up.

However, my mom didn't drop everything as I'd expected. Instead, I could hear her telling my sister, "Shh, you know your father doesn't like us to call it the *curse*."

My ever-sassy sister retorted, "Well he doesn't have *it* does he? How does he know what to call *it*!"

Eventually Mom made her way up to my bedroom carrying with her a mug half full of cold coffee, a pile of clean laundry and the smell of the spaghetti sauce she had been making for dinner. She set the laundry on my bed, and seeing me on the floor with my back to the wall and a storm cloud over my head, she launched into her favourite diversionary tactic. She told me a funny story. By the end of the story she had succeeded in making me laugh. She laughed too and before I knew it we were both holding our sides and laughing that belly laugh that makes you cry. We were laughing and crying over her crazy story, but we were also laughing and crying about me. We cried with the sadness that accompanies the loss of childhood and we laughed with the joy that accompanies nature's miracles.

With this first crisis out of the way, I went to bed a happy girl-woman, not realizing that the trip we were leaving on the next day would bring back the slow burning humiliation and anger. We were going to Cheyenne, Wyoming, a day-long drive from Grand Junction, for a Church Retreat at Saint Somebody's Greek Orthodox Church. I remember sitting in the back of Aunt Connie's big American car next to her son Stevie, who was a freshman in high school, and worrying endlessly that I would "leak" and stain my Levis and the car's dove-grey upholstery. I sniffed the air constantly, worried also that Stevie would be able to smell the blood-soaked pad between my legs. I had noticed that morning that it did kind of smell; the smell had reminded me of the way an emery board smells after you filed your nails. The drive seemed endless.

Upon reaching Cheyenne, I was relieved to find out that we would be staying in a hotel instead of at some unknown Greek person's house. I couldn't bear the thought of disposing of my dirty pads in someone else's trash. We went to the requisite pot luck that night and my sister and I were introduced to lots of "nice Greek boys." Those mothers were relentless matchmakers. We also received instructions from the priest that tomorrow would be a special service which began early in the morning. We were to keep a vow of silence from the time we went to bed that night until we got to church the next morning; the first words we were to speak that day were the words of a hymn that praised God. We practised the hymn a couple of times, took our vow and went back to the hotel.

At the hotel, the argument began over who would sleep with Mimi. My mother thought it was most appropriate that she sleep with my brother and my sister sleep with me. Of course this decision was met with relief by Bruce and dismay by Karen who was sure I would "leak" all over her. I went to bed feeling like a leper. I woke the next morning having ful-

filled Karen's prophecy. I had "leaked" and stained the sheets.
I rushed to the bathroom, and discovered what the expres-
sion "heavy period" meant. My reaction was guttural and
verbal. "Gross!" I shouted venting some of the pent-up frus-
tration I felt. Of course, I woke up the others and my mom
and sister came into the bathroom. They were going through
some kind of pantomime and wouldn't talk to me. I felt confused and angry until I remembered the vow of silence we
had taken the evening before. I had broken my vow! Not
only had I broken my vow, I hadn't even said something
nice. My anger quickly changed to shame. I wondered if
God would forgive me.

Feeling like a failure, I started to take a shower to clean
up. As I was stepping into the tub, my mom thrust at me a
note written on the motel stationery. It read: *It's not good to
get your hair wet when you have your period. You could very
easily catch a cold or even pneumonia. Take a bath.* She turned
off the shower and filled the tub. I submerged myself in
water that quickly turned pink. I felt as if I was cleaning part
of myself only by dirtying the rest of myself. I felt cursed.

At church while the others broke their silence with a
hymn, I sulked. I was beginning to understand what it *meant*
to have a period. It meant you were in a dirty, weakened
state. I thought about my girlfriends who had bragged about
getting their periods. I decided they were brain damaged.

I noticed my mom whispering to Aunt Pauline, the
Sunday School teacher. I saw Aunt Pauline look at me and
then shake her head. Pretty soon my mom leaned to me and

whispered in my ear that I couldn't receive communion because I had my period.

"What?" I said incredulously.

"You can't receive communion," Mom whispered again. "It's supposed to be a bloodless sacrifice and you're bleeding. It's not clean. You are supposed to be pure, that's why you say confession and fast, to purify yourself."

I fumed. If I was so impure why did I have to fast that morning and skip breakfast like everyone else who was receiving communion? Glowering, I sat in the pew while the rest of the congregation received communion. I knew that it was now obvious to everyone in the church that I had the curse. Sitting there in my damp, bulky, diaper-like Kotex with greasy hair I hadn't been allowed to wash that morning, my stomach growling with hunger, I felt sure that everyone looked at me with revulsion as they returned from receiving communion. There was no question in my mind now what it meant to menstruate. I endured the rest of the day by plotting my revolt.

The next morning I took a shower and washed my hair. I locked myself in the bathroom until my sister showed me how to use a tampon. My rebellion was contagious. Pretty soon my sister and I were no longer taking our stained underwear to dry in the privacy of our rooms, but leaving them hanging on the rod in the bathroom in full sight of my brother and dad. We made remarks about having the curse at the dinner table just to see Dad squirm. Not brave enough to actually receive communion while we were menstruating, we made a show of how delicious our breakfast tasted when the rest of our family was fasting. We created a new meaning for our periods; they were now a source of power we could use to make others uncomfortable. Typical teenage behaviour.

Maybe someday I'll get up the nerve to take communion while menstruating. Then again, maybe I won't — I wouldn't want God to take revenge on me by making a large red stain appear on the back of my skirt just as I turn my back on the congregation.

MENSTRUAL MYTH #4

False: You can't get pregnant if you have sex when you've got your period.

Fact: Although it's unusual for pregnancy to happen during menstruation, it has been known to happen.

Sexually active people should always use condoms. They protect you from pregnancy and from sexually transmitted diseases, like HIV/AIDS. Condoms are small latex bags that slide onto the man's erect penis and catch the semen when he ejaculates. They are easily available at drugstores.

TURNINGS

ROSEMARY VOGT

*Rosemary Vogt grew up on a dairy farm on the Prairies
in the 1960s. In "Turnings," Rosemary remembers the
story of her first period. Though farming is hard work,
Rosie has always liked it. It's something she knows how
to do, something that makes her feel grown-up and
confident. When her first period arrives, Rosie is upset
that she has to deal with it alone but she soon realizes
that she knows how to take care of herself.*

"*I* KNOW YOU HATE ME!" I screamed at my mother through
the screen of the bedroom window. She remained silent as
she stooped over to pick fresh lettuce and stuff it into a plastic bag. I continued to stare at her through the window, feeling sick to my stomach with anger.

Only a moment ago my mother had told me on her way
out to the garden that she and Dad were going camping for
a week with her "pal" Linda.

I thought it was so unfair. She had never done anything

like that with me! How could she take Linda away like this and leave me alone at the farm with my brother? It was July and the garden was bursting with produce that needed to be looked after. I was only thirteen!

She came in from the garden but never looked at me. I knew she couldn't; she didn't have the courage to. I stood off to the side of the kitchen and watched her as she went about packing food, and then carried it out to the camper. All the time I was wondering what went through that head of hers. What had I done to her to make her reject me this way? Why did she decide to take her "pal" Linda camping for a week and not me? Linda was seventeen. Did she think I was too young and immature to spend time with? The whole thing hurt my feelings more than I can explain.

The camper was packed with bedding and enough food for a week. I watched it disappear down the country road towards the house where Linda lived four miles away, and with it, my mother, father and eight year old sister.

Standing in the yard in the dim evening light, I felt as though the bottom of my world had just fallen out. She had left me in silence, not spoken a word. There was a silent understanding that I would do whatever needed to be done. I was capable. Although I was only thirteen, I had handled adult responsibilities for a long time. All the times Mother and Dad had been separated, I would cook and clean, bake and run the farm's private milk sales. Even when she was around, I would busy myself with a chore. But always I would keep as far away from her as possible; something about being near her made me uncomfortable. Yet somehow I was jealous of Linda for being with her instead of me! I couldn't understand my feelings.

Just last summer Mom had whipped me twice real bad for reasons I still did not understand. Although I had tried to forget, the events suddenly came back into my head. It had been mid-afternoon, and both times she had grabbed me by the hair, led me to the car, and threw me into the back seat. At first I didn't know where she was taking me but soon it was obvious that she was heading for an old vacant house on another farm my father owned. Once inside the old house, she whipped me with a thin telephone cord. No words were spoken. The second time it happened I thought that she would kill me with that cord and wondered who would find me in that old house and how my death would be explained.

Now I stood in the semi-darkness, under the yard light. Hands deep inside my blue jeans pockets, I gazed at the long shadow my body created on the ground. Through the kitchen window, I could see Jerry at the table eating his night snack of Rice Krispies cereal. I wanted my life to make sense but it didn't. I began to walk. Across the yard, to the end of the driveway, then west to Highway 59, a quarter mile away.

As I passed the big fresh haystack of alfalfa, I remembered the day that I had cooked for all the hired men. With the threat of rain, Dad had been in a hurry to get the bales

off the field. We always provided food for the workers. It had
been me frying up the hamburgers, mashing the potatoes
and dishing out huge portions of fresh chocolate cake and
ice cream.

It was a beautiful clear summer evening on the prairie.
The frogs croaked their evening prayers and the birds sang
out softly. It was such a contrast to the chaos inside me. I
had never yelled at my mother before. Somehow the words
"I know you hate me" just came out of my mouth. I had not
been able to stop them. It was so out of character; I was
always quiet and never spoke out of turn.

Reaching the highway, I sat down in the ditch. I wanted
to run away but where would I go? If I went north, the highway would take me to Winnipeg. I doubted Uncle Jake and
Auntie Irma would be very pleased about me living with
them. If I went south, I'd go past the beach where my mother and Linda were camping, and eventually end up in North
Dakota. They'd never let me cross the border on foot. I had
no choice but to go back to that farm and finish growing up
so I could get away.

The sound of a motor bike brought me back to reality.
Looking up over my shoulder, I saw my brother Jerry. "Get
over here!" he said in his sternest voice. "What do you think
you're doing out here anyway?" I knew he was right and,
feeling very foolish, I climbed up on the bike behind him.

The next morning I was awakened by Jerry's shouting to
hurry and get out of bed. The cattle were out of the pasture
and he needed my help to get them back in. Quickly I

pulled on a pair of jeans and a T-shirt, ran a brush through my hair, then bounded down the stairs and out of the house.

The cattle were already all over the lawn, the garden, the ditches and the road. A few greedy cows were feasting on fresh alfalfa bales beside the barn. I shook my head — it looked so hopeless. How would the two of us ever round up all those cattle? Jerry was over at the road now, keeping a small group from straying any further. I ran around the back of the house to the garden, knowing they would be after the corn. Walking unseen behind the lilac bushes I came out between the corn and the barbed wire fence, frightening the cattle out of the garden and back towards the gate where our faithful dogs were on guard.

Worried about Jerry, I started to run towards the road. I felt cramps in my lower stomach and, thinking it was from running too hard, slowed down to a fast walk. Jerry was moving the cows toward the gate. Bridget and Sparky kept those inside the gate from coming out again. Everything looked as though it was under control. This was my opportunity to run inside to the bathroom. The cramps were really bothering me.

Breathlessly I pulled down my jeans and sat on the toilet. I gasped and my eyes opened wide at the sight of bloodstains on my underwear. I began to shake, my head spinning. Had I run too hard or what?

Then reality set in. I realized that I had my first period. Of all the times to get my first period! Here I was at home alone with my older brother, my mother busy at the beach bonding with Linda. I would make her pay; she would be sorry. One way or another I would pay her back for all the hurt and neglect. I would shut her out of my life forever. I would never tell her, I decided. My periods would be my very own secret.

"Rooooosie!" I heard Jerry calling me. I knew he needed my help.

I grabbed some toilet paper, rolled it up and stuffed it into my underwear. Then I pulled up my pants and hurried to my mother's room to look for pads. Sure enough I found some in her closet. Grabbing the box, I ran upstairs to where I had the brand new sanitary belt the school health nurse had given out to the grade seven girls. Awkwardly I put the pad in place and climbed into the sanitary belt, wondering how to attach the long tabs of pad to the belt.

"Roooosie!"

Oh Jerry, shut up already! I thought. Surely he would be wondering why I was taking so long to come back outside to help him. There was no way I was going to try to explain this to him!

Satisfied that the pad and belt were secured, I pulled my soiled underwear back up. It felt wet and uncomfortable. I wanted to take a bath but knew I'd have to wait until later.

I hurried out to the yard. Jerry was having a problem with a few stubborn cows. He looked at me disapprovingly, and said, "Where were you?"

I didn't answer. I was thinking of how uncomfortable the bulky pad felt between my legs and how irritating the belt felt in the crack of my bottom. As we rounded up the last of the stray cows, I hoped Jerry would not see the bulge of the pad in my jeans. Occasionally I felt a gush of liquid from my body and more cramps. So many thoughts were going through my head. I had not imagined that the "flow" would be so heavy. Would it always be this way? How long would it last? Should I take something for the cramps?

With the last of the cows behind the fence, I helped Jerry swing over the long gate and secure the latch. I knew that we would have to go check the fence later to see where the cows had escaped. Jerry headed for the barn to begin the chores and I went to the house.

Once inside, I ran the bathwater and went about collecting clean underwear, clothing and pads. I wondered about blood in the bathwater. I remembered the health nurse telling us that the flow would stop in the water. Locking the bathroom door, I began to undress. I removed the heavily soiled pad and wrapped it in toilet paper and hid it deep inside the waste basket. I stepped into the tub and slowly sat down. The water around me turned red! I remained frozen for a few seconds and then swished the water with my hands and the redness disappeared. I was relieved. I washed myself all over and stepped out of the tub.

As I dried myself off, the towel became stained with blood. How quickly the flow began again! I grabbed some toilet paper and stuffed it between my legs, then fumbled with getting a pad in place and attached to the sanitary belt. I realized the tabs on the pad were longer than necessary and that I would have to do some experimenting to get the pad secure and comfortable. The back tab was the hardest to do and no matter where I placed the pad and belt, it always ended up in the crack of my bottom. I would just have to get used to it like all other women did.

Once I was dressed, I let the water out of the tub and saw to my surprise little clots of blood in the water. Again I wondered if this was normal; the health nurse had said nothing about clots of blood. I hid the box of pads behind a bunch of towels in the cupboard and wondered how long they would last. I would have to figure out a way to get Jerry to take me to town.

As I walked to the kitchen, I felt the awkwardness of the bulky pad between my legs. No matter how I moved, it felt fat and conspicuous. I walked to the dining room, the livingroom and back to the kitchen sink and stood by the window.

Looking out across the yard it was hard to picture the chaos of the scattered cattle earlier that morning. Everything had changed. I had grown and matured — I could feel it! It didn't seem to matter any more about Mom and Linda camping. I had my period now; I was a woman. I found pads, figured out the sanitary belt. I felt wise, mature, feminine.

In that moment as I stood by the window, I imagined that the farm was mine and that Jerry in the barn doing the chores was my hired man. I would eat breakfast, then bake a fresh chocolate cake. Then I would go to the milk house to sterilize jars for fresh milk for our private customers.

Life would go on and no one would ever know the events of the day except me.

If you or a person you know is being abused by an adult the way that Rosie was by her mother, it's important to know that nobody has to put up with this kind of treatment. There are people out there that can help you deal with it. Talk to someone you trust or call the KIDS HELP LINE at 1-800-668-6868 (in Canada); the YOUTH CRISIS HOTLINE at 1-800-448-4663 (in the United States); or the CHILDLINE at 0800-1111 (in Britain). Some challenges in life are just too big for one person to handle alone.

MENSTRUAL MYTH #5

False: Virgins can't use tampons.

Fact: Virgins can use tampons. If you want, you can use a tampon the very first time you menstruate.

People think this myth is true because of the hymen, the thin membrane that protects your vaginal opening when you're young. Inserting a tampon may stretch this membrane. Any young woman who rides bikes or horses, does gymnastics or is very physically active has likely stretched open her hymen by the time of her first period. You might be able to see your hymen if you look at your vaginal opening in a mirror. The hymen will be the light pink skin at the opening of your vagina. If it's been stretched open, you'll see holes in it or it'll look like a ragged ring of pink skin.

THE PASSAGE

*Some people, like the women described in the stories
that follow, believe that a girl's first period is very special
and that it deserves celebration. They see getting
your first period as a wonderful gift that
marks a girl's passage into a new stage of life.*

*You can make your own period a special time by
celebrating it with your friends and your family or
celebrating it by yourself in a secret way. While getting your
period may not transform you overnight, it's like a sign that
points you in a new direction.*

NEW MOON

LILIAN NATTEL

*Author Lilian Nattel has set her story in a village in
Poland in the 1890s. Misha, a young Jewish woman,
has her first period. Girls in the village get their periods
late and marry as young as fourteen or fifteen, so first
menstruation signals that a young woman is ready to
start a family of her own. Misha comes from a long line
of women healers and midwives, and her mother
celebrates the event by sharing this female history.*

WHEN MISHA GOT HER FIRST period, she knew what to
expect. The girls talked, and she wasn't ashamed to ask her
mother. "If you're old enough to ask, you're old enough to
know," her mother used to say.

With her mother's help, Misha had prepared monthly
cloths, the strips of clean cotton rags that she could pin to her
underthings when she had her period. And after she fixed
herself up, she went to find her mother in the root cellar.

The cellar door was open and Misha climbed down slowly,

as befit her new dignity, moving from light into darkness.
The smell of hay baking in the sun gave way to the smell of
moist earth, and there was a moment of blindness until her
eyes adjusted to the cellar dusk. Her mother wore a wide
apron embroidered with red thread, and in the muted light,
it seemed to float as her mother reached up to hang a basket.

Already a head taller than her mother, Misha bent to
lean her head on her mother's shoulder, feeling strangely shy.
She whispered, "Mama, I'm not a child any more."

Her mother didn't slap her face, as was the custom.
Instead she put an arm around Misha's waist and stroked her
hair.

When a girl first got her period, most mothers would
slap her across the face: a superstition, supposed to keep
away bad spirits. But Misha's mother, a midwife, helped all
the women of the village bring their babies into the world.
She was an herbalist, too, preparing medicines from the
plants and flowers in the woods. Misha's mother was not
afraid of spirits.

"May the Holy One be praised that I lived until today,"
Misha's mother said. "Now I have something to give you.
Come, my dear," she said, taking Misha's hand.

When they came upstairs, Misha looked curiously
around the room they'd shared so long wondering what there
could possibly be within these four corners that she hadn't
looked under and over and behind a hundred times. There
was the table, and the bench, and the stove, the braids of
garlic and onions and drying mushrooms, the shelves of

dishes and cups and jars, the big cooking pot, and the clay
bowls, the landscape her grandmother had embroidered with
its elephants in blue-tasseled cloths, the braided rag rug
beside the bed she shared with her mother.

"Misha," her mother said. "You're sixteen years old and a
woman now. I'm giving you the key to the bridal trunk that
your father made for you, and I hope that you'll fill it with
good things. Come here child, and let me show you what's
inside so when I'm gone you remember what you need to."
Her mother moved the brass candlesticks, the wooden bowl
and the red woolen shawl that had covered the trunk for so
long, Misha had forgotten that it was anything but a shelf or
a bench.

Lifting the lid of the trunk, her mother took out a folded
cloth. "This was my mother's," she said, "whom you were
named for. She made it before I was born."

As she pulled back an edge of the cloth, Misha saw the
carefully detailed stitching of leaves, flowers and roots. "Tansy,
hellebore, bryony, belladonna," Misha named the plants with
delight. "And this one?" She pointed to a bell-shaped rose and
purple flower, its inside speckled with red dots.

"Foxglove," her mother said, unfurling the finely spun
cloth so that it lay shimmering across the floor between
them. "Very strong for the heart. Your grandmother hung
this cloth over my cradle when I was born. I did the same,
and it protected you until you could walk." Her finger traced
the delicate threads. "Every one of these flowers is strong and
dangerous."

"I know," Misha said. What she didn't mention to her mother was that she had made various remedies from these plants, testing them on her cat. The cat was not very grateful for Misha's interest, but luckily had survived.

"It's not the strongest plants that are the best for everything. At the right time, something as simple as raspberry leaf tea can do more good. You'd find out for yourself if you were helping me. You could start tomorrow — if you want to."

Misha had been waiting a long time for her mother to begin training her to be a midwife. "Tomorrow's good," she said.

Next her mother took from the trunk a hair wreath plaited like the braids of a round Sabbath bread, fair and dark and russet coloured, and in the centre a lock of moon-white hair. "All the women in the family, when their hair is cut after the wedding, braid a lock into this, so that their daughters won't forget them."

"And this one?" Misha asked, touching the lock in the centre.

"My grandmother's. Her hair was always white, she told me, even when she was a girl younger than you."

Misha saw with great interest how the white hair in the centre set off the other braids like the moon rising above a newly ploughed field, the browns and blacks of the earth rich in its glow. How soft the white hair looked, but just as she reached out a finger to touch it, her mother returned the wreath to the trunk.

"Is there anything of yours, Mama?"

"Of course," she said lightly, picking up a silk-wrapped bundle. "My family's wedding gift."

"That was your dowry?" Misha asked in astonishment as she looked at what her mother held.

"Well, the silver candlesticks I brought with me were ugly. My Papa was proud. The candlesticks were heavy. Everything he owned was in them. But so ugly. I begged your father to sell them. I wanted him to make something for me himself. Something beautiful." Tenderly she put the wooden carving with its large round base into Misha's hands. "Feel how smooth." Misha ran her fingers across the carving. A winged figure was blowing a ram's horn, its head tilted back. And out of the horn, tiny leaves and flowers curled upward and around the rim, climbing the point of a wing. "You see?" Her mother put a key into the back of the base and turned. Music cascaded from the horn. Misha recognized the song. "*Ani maamin,*" she sang softly, "I believe in the coming of the Messiah, even though he may tarry, I believe."

"There's one more thing," her mother said. She took out a silver box with ivory inlay. "This belonged to my great-grandmother, Blema. I was named for her. In her day, she was the women's prayer-leader, and she kept the prayers in this box."

In synagogue, men and women sat separately, men downstairs and women up in the balcony. The women, unable to understand the Hebrew prayers that the men chanted below, followed their prayer-leader, a woman who recited their own unique prayers in the language they spoke every day: Yiddish.

Misha lifted the lid of the box. Inside was a parchment-thin pamphlet. It was the prayer for the New Moon, the first day of the Hebrew month.

"Now that you're a woman," her mother said, "on the New Moon you'll pray with the women."

Every month on *Rosh Hodesh,* the New Moon, the women celebrated together. It was a woman's holiday, a day of rest from sewing and cooking. In the evening they would gather to sing, to pray for the well-being of their family and friends, and to thank the Holy One for all their blessings. Afterward, they would eat cake and talk — how they would talk!

"I hope the cake's good," Misha said.

"Only the best," her mother answered.

So Misha would join the women on the New Moon. She would stand with her mother in the candle light, their voices blending as they sang. Afterward, the young married women, just a year or two older than Misha, would huddle with the girls, whispering and laughing. And even the old women, the grandmothers, would have something to tell about how things were, and how they could be.

MOON MOVEMENTS

The words "menstruate" and "menses" come from the Latin word *mensis* which means "month." The ancient Romans, whose language was Latin, based their months on the moon's cycle of twenty-eight days. Women were thought to have a special relationship with the moon because their menstrual cycle followed a pattern similar in length to the moon's phases.

Many other cultures have also noticed that the moon's phases and a woman's menstrual cycle are sometimes the same. In different folk stories, mythologies and religions, the moon is thought to be female. From ancient times right up to the present day, women have named their menstrual flow "moontime" or "moonflowers" to show this relationship between the moon and a woman's body.

Stories are told that women were able to control the time of their bleeding through prayers to the full moon. Some women in ancient times believed that they had spiritual power when all the women of their community were able to menstruate at the same time. If a woman menstruated out of time with the other members of her group, she would sit in the light of the full moon to bring her cycle back into synchronicity with the others. Some women still practise this ancient tradition today.

(cont'd)

Studies done by scientists show that ancient cultures knew what they were talking about. These studies show that menstrual cycles are indeed affected by the amount of natural light a woman experiences. However, it seems that many women have lost their relationship with the moon because they live in cities that are brightly lit at night or because they stay indoors much more than women of earlier societies. Even so, a woman may still find that her periods follow the phases of the moon.

Some scientists are unsure about a connection between the moon and a woman's body. But is it really so surprising? We humans, like plants and animals, have a relationship to the planet that we live on. The moon's phases affect the ocean tides. Wouldn't these phases also affect our bodies?

Watch a calendar of moon phases to see what pattern your cycle follows. Then you might be able to tell when your period is due just by looking at the night sky!

MY BODY IS MY TEMPLE

IDA FISHER

*In this story, Ida Fisher shares the warm memories of
her family's celebration of womanhood. When Ida gets
her first period, the women of her family give her gifts,
helpful advice and even a party with her favourite
foods. Ida learns to respect her body and
all it has to teach her.*

MY FIRST MENSTRUAL FLOW was a time for celebration in our
matriarchal family. "Now you can make babies," my mother
exclaimed. She had a gentle understanding smile on her lips.
She hugged and kissed me, indicating I had done something
right. I was pampered for the rest of the day. Yet upon waking that July morning, I had been horrified at the mess in
my pyjamas. Splotches of dark blood stained my bedclothes.
I washed my body as if it was a stranger to me; it had let me
down. Was I dying?

I knew there would be changes in my body that summer of 1952. I knew I needed to be at the cottage with loved ones. In early April, I had refused to go to camp. I didn't understand why I did not want to go. Mother tried to persuade me, but I knew I had to be at the family cottage.

I had seen a movie in health class in the spring. Miss Barnett, the Phys Ed teacher, said she felt "uncomfortable talking to us" so she invited Mrs Fealth, the public health nurse, into our all-girl class to answer "personal questions." Mrs Fealth talked about menses as if it was going to be a sweet sixteen party. She showed us this Walt Disney movie depicting the eggs and sperm as little fish swimming together happily. She said, "Once you flow every twenty-eight days, you will be physically ready to conceive." She used lots of jargon I did not understand, but I was too embarrassed to ask questions. I figured all my classmates knew more than I. She talked about intercourse, fallopian tubes, the penis and testes as if we were all medical students. If she had used locker-room words like "screw" and "prick," I probably would have understood.

When I finally asked my question, she responded, "You do not get pregnant every time you have sex." What a great idea, I thought. I was glad she had come to class that day.

The fateful Sunday summer morning of my first blood, Mother drove me to the drugstore in the village. Thank goodness it was open. On the way, I saw life a little differently. The flowers with pistils and stamens seemed closer to me. Tiny pine cones on the roadside had new significance. The "eggs for sale" sign on the local farmhouse had new meaning. Life force sprang up everywhere. I was glad to be a woman and glad to be alive.

The male pharmacist had a funny look in his eyes when my mother stood by me and asked politely, "One box of blue Kotex, a belt, safety pins and a box of fragrant dusting powder." Then she hugged me right in the store and said, "I am so proud of you, all grown up and everything."

We rushed home with our purchases. I was carefully instructed how to use this new equipment. It sure was different than the movie version. I preened when the thick white pad was firmly ensconced. I was a woman, I breathed to myself. Yet the pad was bulky and uncomfortable. The pins stuck directly into my lower abdomen. I did not feel grown up.

Mother told me, "Never be embarrassed about buying Kotex from a man in the drugstore. It is the most natural thing in the world, just like toothpaste." That was fine to say, Mother, but I always felt every male druggist relished the moment when a young woman would shyly ask for the "unmentionables." For the next forty years I was to feel that flush of femininity. Thank heavens Tampax and self-serve stores came into being.

That day my mother tried to teach me the proper names for the private parts of my body, but at twelve years old, I had trouble remembering the difference between *vagina* and *uterus.* I just knew I had one of each and some day it would all make sense.

My grandmother was to be informed of this most important event. Dressed in a white sunsuit, I was carted to her house — feeling like Little Red Riding Hood without the basket — and I was proudly shown off. Grandma grinned, "Your body is your temple, forever. You must care for and clean your temple as carefully as a high priestess. You are responsible for what happens in your temple. Now you can make babies. Always remember, my dear, it is your temple." She handed me a ten dollar bill which was to help me forget the pains in my lower abdomen. I was kissed and hugged and told to be good.

Auntie Ruth, my favourite aunt, was next on the list, and I didn't mind being whisked off to her cottage. She was right on the beach. The three of us walked hand in hand along the hot sand. My mother told her the news. Auntie Ruth jumped for joy. She ran into the waves and danced around. She shrieked with enthusiasm, "My dear, my dear, you are a woman now. Nothing can take you back to childhood. The miracle of love can bring you babies. You must be very careful whom you love. Don't let just anyone touch you or love you. Even be careful when you play Spin-the-Bottle. You are a lady now. Babies come easily. Be very careful." She scooped up a handful of water right from the lake and sprinkled fresh water on my head. She presented me with her cherished basket which she carried to the beach. I was a woman.

Proud of my matriarchal inheritance, I was a debutante, emerging from childhood. The celebration continued. I needed the recognition of the females in my family. Mother

made my favourite dinner that night: baked Idaho potatoes
and rare steak barbecued on the new outdoor brick grill.
Cousins and aunties were invited and each brought me a
feminine token: a wild flower bouquet from Aunt Flora, a
poetry book by Elizabeth Barrett Browning from Aunt Rose,
a box of Dutch chocolates from Mora and a painted silk
scarf from Dorothy. Smiled upon from above, I was loved by
my women relatives.

This day was the beginning of a new person in our family circle. My monthlies came regularly without aggravation
or pain. I was never "cursed" with any menstrual problems.
Now, forty-one years later, I wonder if the gentle and warm
initiation given to me by my family had anything to do with
my easy menstrual cycles.

A REMARKABLE FACT

Women have an organ that's for pleasure only. It's
called the clitoris. This tiny bud-shaped organ is
located outside your body at the top of your labia.
You can barely see it when it isn't aroused, but you
can probably feel a warm, pleasant sensation when
you rub this area gently. Experiment! Very few other
animal species (and only females!) have a clitoris —
just a few kinds of monkeys and humans are lucky
enough.

PAP SMEARS AND PELVIC EXAMINATIONS

Pelvic exams and pap smears are how women protect themselves from dangerous internal illnesses like cancer, or infections like yeast and sexually transmitted diseases. If infections are allowed to grow for too long, a woman may become *infertile* (not able to have babies) and will get very sick. Because our reproductive organs are mainly inside, it's difficult to know if everything is healthy.

You should have a pelvic exam and pap smear if you have been menstruating for a few years, if you're sexually active, or if you notice anything unusual with your menstrual blood, your cycle or your daily secretions. Most women have these exams done about once a year.

This is what happens during a pelvic exam: The doctor or nurse practitioner will have you undress from the waist down. You'll get to wear a special gown or be given a sheet to cover yourself. Then the doctor will have you lie down on a medical bed. You will spread your legs and put your feet up in *stirrups* (metal holders) so that the doctor will have a good clear view of your vulva. Using an instrument called a *speculum* and jelly for lubricant, the doctor will open up your vagina. She'll look inside to see that things are a nice healthy colour and that your cervix looks right. She'll have rubber gloves on and she'll

(cont'd)

slide two fingers inside to feel that your ovaries and uterus have no unusual bumps. She may press your belly too to feel your uterus and ovaries from that angle.

A pap smear happens during the pelvic exam. The doctor will insert a long cotton swab into your vagina up to your cervix. This will pick up a "smear" of the secretions and cells of the cervix. The swab is taken to a lab and looked at to see if there is anything unusual. If you are sexually active, tell the doctor and she will also test for common sexually transmitted diseases.

Be sure to tell your doctor all about your menstrual cycle. Try to remember when you last had your period and how long your periods last. If there's anything unusual, tell the doctor about it. Ask your doctor any questions you have. This is your body and you need to know everything there is to know about it!

You may feel nervous about your pelvic exam. Try breathing deeply, think relaxing thoughts and remember that most adult women do this at least once every year. If you're really nervous, your tense muscles may cause some discomfort. You might want your mom or someone else close to you to come with you for the first time. If this is your first pelvic exam, tell the doctor — she will talk you through it.

Mom and Me and the Sisters of the Assumption

GERMAINE ST. PAUL

*It doesn't take much to make your first period a special
time. Germaine St. Paul still remembers getting her first
period while she was living away from home in a
Catholic boarding school. The nuns or "sisters" who
ran the school celebrated the event with quiet
but warm recognition.*

THE SUMMER BEFORE I TURNED eleven, my mother told me
about menstruation.

Mom was sitting at her electric sewing machine (a novelty in the early 1950s) and I was sitting on the floor beside
her, reading comics. She told me that when a girl reached my
age or older, her body began preparing to make babies. Mom

said that each month a girl's womb would prepare a sort of nest for a baby to grow in and this nest was made mostly of blood. The nest of blood always had to be fresh and so a woman's body would get rid of this blood if there was no baby in it. This happened every month, she said, about the same time each month, every twenty-eight days or so. This time in a woman's month was called "menstruation," but that was the medical name and most women called it a "period." Mom also said that some women called it "the curse" but as the beginning of menstruation was a sign that a girl was becoming a woman, Mom didn't think it was a curse. As we sat there together with the sunlight and a delicate breeze both streaming through the open window, I felt that my Mom was so special and that now I was special too because of what she had said.

Mom also explained about pads. As far as I can recall, there were only Kotex and Modess pads then. Tampax was new and not to be used by me, said Mom; that was just for married ladies. The Modess ads in magazines were a full-page picture of a beautiful woman in a long formal dress with the words "Modess. To be sure." Now I finally knew what that meant! Mom showed me a "sanitary belt" — something like a garter belt with two garter-like loops of metal, one on each end, that the ends of the "sanitary pad" were hooked into — and showed me how to wear the belt and pad.

I was going to be living in a Roman Catholic convent that school year. Mom told me that nuns, being women, also menstruated. If I were at the convent when I began to have periods, I was to tell a nun and she would know how to help me.

And so it came to pass. The stain in my panties happened that winter — I noticed it when undressing for bed one night. I told one of the nuns and she gave me a few home-made pads of layered, folded white cotton, a home-made sanitary belt also made of white cotton, and two safety pins. I told her I knew how to put them on and I did so. This menstruation material was all reused after being deposited in special laundry baskets and bleached and washed back to whiteness in the convent's basement laundry. Then Sister told me that, just for that one night, I could stay up until the oldest girls went to bed because I was becoming a woman. So I sat in a study room and read a book until it was the older girls' bedtime.

I felt very adult being able to stay up late. The study room was fairly small and the door was left open. There was no one but me in the room and the convent was very quiet. During the time I was there, every nun in the convent came by to greet me and to say good night. The evening took on a ritual quality, with each nun coming in, those whom I didn't know well introducing themselves to me, each of them saying a few words and leaving, and a few minutes later another one arriving, her long skirts swishing quietly. Thus, remembering my first period invokes in me a feeling of pride and a warm sense of belonging to the sisterhood of women.

THE PILL AND MENSTRUATION

The birth control pill, often just called The Pill, is a mixture of artificial hormones. The Pill tells your body that it doesn't need to ovulate. A woman takes a birth control pill each day for twenty-one days and then takes a "sugar pill" for seven days (or no pills at all) and has her period. She then begins the cycle again, taking a pill each day for another twenty-one days. While many women take The Pill to prevent pregnancy, doctors sometimes put young women on it to help regulate their periods and ease very painful menstrual cramps. It can work wonders.

However, the hormone system of our bodies is very complicated and scientists don't fully understand all the effects of hormones. Sometimes women on The Pill gain weight (fluid not fat), have light bleeding between their periods, lose their sex drive, or become more susceptible to certain kinds of cancer (especially if they are smokers). If you're thinking of using The Pill, try to learn as much as you can about the medication before you make the choice. If you know any female relatives who've used The Pill, you may want to ask them about their experiences. Health clinics and teen clinics have brochures that explain The Pill in detail as well as helpful staff that can answer your questions.

BREASTS

Breasts come in all sorts of shapes and sizes. Even your own two breasts will be different shapes and sizes, with the left one probably being a little larger than the right. *This is normal!* Sometimes women grow hair around their nipples, just like men do. Nipples may stick out or stick in and will vary in colour from woman to woman. All this is normal too. To estimate the shape and size of your future breasts, look at your mother and aunts and other female relatives.

Your breast size and tenderness will vary slightly with your menstrual cycle because, like your reproductive organs and so much else of you, breasts also respond to hormones. Your breasts might feel fuller and tender at the time of ovulation and menstruation. For some women, the first signs of pregnancy are felt in the breasts, which become swollen.

Get familiar with your breasts. Check with your mother or doctor about breast examinations. A breast examination is an easy procedure you can do in the shower to feel for unusual lumps that may be cancerous. Breasts are naturally lumpy and it's important to learn which lumps are normal. Lumps that are normal will change with your menstrual cycle. You can help reduce normal breast lumps by cutting back on fat, caffeine, alcohol and salt in your diet, and by not smoking.

PUTTING IT
ALL TOGETHER

*So much happens around the time of your first period.
What does it all mean? Sometimes menstruation gives you
insight into other aspects of life. Sometimes your period just
makes life seem all the more complicated. In this last section
of stories, young women try to make sense of it all. Maybe
they'll help you figure some things out too.*

LEARNING ABOUT JEELY JARS

LOUISE SIMON

*Sometimes your period can bring you the feeling that
you're seeing things the way they really are for the very
first time. Jenny, the main character in Louise Simon's
story, lives on a ranch in Alberta. She begins menstruating while her mother and father are away from home.
The event makes her think about life in a new light,
especially about the confusing and sometimes unhappy
relations between men and women.*

JENNY SLEPT IN BECAUSE she had forgotten to set the alarm.
Her brother Evan didn't call her before he went off to milk
the cows, water stock and do those other before-school
chores.

The whole problem had begun the night before when
she stayed up late reading. If her father had been home this
wouldn't have happened. He expected her in bed by ten and

would probably have nixed the book. It was the kind of book her mother also would have said was too old for her.

Jenny had discovered the novel on the top shelf of the school library. She'd become completely absorbed with the main character, an awful, warped man who dominated and terrified his wife and children. He was contemptuous of all of them but his youngest daughter, the clever one. He had counted on her to win the school prize and had boasted about it to the whole town. He nagged her endlessly to keep at her books. When she failed to win she hung herself. Now Jenny remembered what had jerked her awake — her dream of a young girl's body swinging from a rope in their kitchen. In the dream, Jenny had backed into the body, and she could still feel the sensation of it touching her as she awoke.

She had to get the whole story out of her mind and dress quickly for school. It was already 8:15. They should be leaving in a few minutes. It was then she discovered the blood-stain on her bloomers. It was what her mother had told her would happen. Fortunately the bloomers were navy. The stain would never show. The only advantage she could think of for the ugly things...

She rummaged in her dresser drawer for the elastic belt her mother had given her during the talk. Her mother had also provided a box of those pads, thick as mattresses. She could hear her mother's voice lecturing: "Rest as much as possible for a couple of days when your period starts. Don't get cold and don't talk about it to the other girls at school. Let me know when it happens." Her mother just assumed she'd never talk about this to any boy, even her brother, and probably she wouldn't.

But now her mother was away, staying in a boarding house in town where she'd be close to the doctor and the hospital. She'd been there for the past month waiting to have a baby. She told Jenny she wouldn't have too much difficulty keeping house for just her father and Evan. And her father was in town too, visiting her mother.

Oh well, her mother always over-dramatized things, thought Jenny. There, she got the ends of the damned pad stuck in the little metal hitches like a harness. She hoped it wouldn't show under her favourite skirt which fit so well. She just had to wear that skirt because Evan had told her some of the men would be over today to work the stock. That meant Shammy might be coming. She'd hoped they'd still be here when school was dismissed.

She ran downstairs just as her brother walked in with a pail of milk, bubbles floating on top. She helped him strain it, then covered it and put it in the pantry.

"Come on. We'll have to run to get to school in time. And the creek's rising." He pulled her by the hand but she hung back.

"Just a sec, Evie, I'll grab some bread and jam." Her mother would have been horrified with that sort of breakfast.

They ran all the way, Jenny trying to gobble her breakfast. Yes, the creek was high, but they could still cross on the footbridge. She loved the way the fast-moving brown water flowed under it, intent on getting somewhere else. As they raced across the last stretch, they could see the kids all lined up at the entrance to the school. The teacher saw them coming and waited until, panting, they stood in line. Then she marched them all inside.

School didn't go particularly well. It wasn't the best part of Jenny's day at any time. And today the teacher had filled two blackboards with history notes for her to copy. She loathed history, and copying notes she'd have to memorize later was an awful chore. She and Evan were both in high school now and the teacher of the one-room school didn't have much time to spend with them. Jenny's eyes grew heavy as she scribbled.

She was aware, too, of an unpleasant draggy feeling in her tummy. She could think of no way to relieve it. At recess she felt dull, unwilling to take part in softball, a game she usually loved.

"What's the matter with you, Jenny? It's your turn at bat." Mary Meier was beside her.

"I don't feel too good, Mary."

Mary, older than Jenny, gave her a sharp look. "You've got your period, haven't you?"

Jenny was horrified that she'd guessed, yet strangely comforted too, as though she had become part of some female world she previously had no idea existed.

"Yes, it's my first."

"Your first! Well, you know you'll have to be careful now. You could have a baby."

"How could I have a baby?" What hadn't her mother told her?

"Dummy, if you're with a boy. See, doing this," Mary made a circle with her left forefinger and thumb and plunged the forefinger of her other hand back and forth through the circle. She laughed loudly as she ran off to take her place on first base.

Jenny, her face hot, felt foolish that Mary knew something she didn't. She remembered the hateful father in the book, who, with repugnance to his sick wife, said something like: "You're as much good to me as an empty jeely jar." A jelly jar. She'd wondered about his meaning when she read that; now she felt a sort of uneasy understanding. She found herself thinking about her father and mother too, now that her mother was waiting to have her baby.

It was a relief when school was over and they were all able to escape. The section of the creek running by below the schoolhouse had flooded its banks. Evie, who was checking the situation, reported: "We're going to have to walk around by the main bridge."

They had started out with long strides, when down the side of the north hill rode the young men they were expecting at the ranch. The men were needed to round up mares and their colts for branding. They all passed Jenny and Evan with whoops as they galloped off to the schoolhouse except for Bill, who was Evan's best friend. Jenny, knowing they were going to visit the young teacher, felt a pang because Shammy was with them.

Bill rode along with Jenny and Evan, talking mostly with Evan.

"You kids don't have to walk around. I'll ride you across on Baby here."

"That's great, Bill. How's Baby gonna behave with someone in a skirt behind the saddle?" Jenny knew the horses that the men rode weren't always that tame.

"Oh, she'll be fine," assured Bill. Evan helped Jenny get seated behind Bill with her skirt pulled up. "Just don't kick her sides — she always bucks if we try that."

They'd reached the creek and started across what had become a fast-flowing river, deeper than they expected. To keep her shoes dry, Jenny bent her legs back against Baby's flanks. When they were on dry ground again Baby started bucking. Jenny tumbled off, landing awkwardly on her right shoulder.

"Are you okay?" Peering down, Bill looked worried.

"Oh, I'm fine." Jenny scrambled to her feet trying to look casual, as though that was her usual method of dismounting. "Thanks for the lift, Bill. You've saved us a long walk." She smiled up at him despite her numb shoulder, feeling utterly clumsy. Slinking off toward the house, she didn't wait to see if Evan made the trip across. Evan caught up to her.

"Are you sure you weren't hurt? That looked like a bad fall."

"It's my right shoulder," she confessed. "My arm feels useless. But it should be okay soon."

"Bill says the guys won't be doing round-up today. Too much trouble with the colts in deep water."

"Good, there'll just be us for supper." She could prepare something easy for the two of them.

But as she approached the house Jenny noticed someone at the back door. As she came closer she saw it was old Jimmy Larsen sitting on the big stone doorstep. Jimmy roamed around the community and didn't seem to have a home of his own. He'd stop here for a few days, maybe do a few chores, sleep in the hayloft, then be off again to some other neighbour. When her father was here, Jimmy would tell him stories about other people he'd visited. Her father seemed to listen. Jenny knew he must talk about them too.

"You'll stay for supper?" She tried to sound neighbourly like her mother. Old Jimmy seemed glad to scuttle in and settle in a chair by the big Quebec heater where Evan was busy getting a fire going.

"We won't need the kitchen stove. I'll just boil some potatoes and poach eggs for supper. I can manage that I'm sure. And we can have that rice pudding with raisins I put in the pantry last night for dessert." Her arm was feeling better.

Evan set the table on the worn oilcloth before hurrying out to attend to the animals. Jenny had everything going properly on the stove. She set the plates on the back of the stove before she drained the potatoes. The eggs looked cooked, the whites nicely solidified in the big frying pan.

She fetched the platter and the egg-lifter. Holding the platter with her left hand, she lifted the eggs onto it one by one, with her right arm giving her no trouble. Old Jimmy crouched nearby, watching her intently. Confidently she transferred the platter of eggs to her right hand to set it on the plates. That's when the arm went. The platter, twisting in her hand, tilted to one side. She watched helplessly as the eggs slid off the platter into the coal scuttle, the yokes breaking, spreading over chunks of coal. Jimmy Larsen sat tittering like an idiot.

She was outside, sobbing beside the watering trough, blowing her nose furiously, when Evan returned from the barn. She tried to compose herself but gaspy sobs still heaved up from her chest. She told him what had happened, told him about Old Jimmy.

"Come on, I'm hungry. Why do you mind an old man who is silly in his head?" Evan sounded exasperated even as he handed her his not-too-clean hanky. Evan was older than Jenny. When their parents were away he was considered to be in charge. He was usually more like a good friend but he had little patience with her when she cried.

She scooped water up from the trough, splashing her face and then wiping it with his handkerchief. She could do nothing about her red eyes. She hated going back into the house with that old man there and longed just to walk down to the creek, to listen to the rush of the flood and hear the slap of willow branches in the high water.

Returning to the dining room, she found Evan had already put eggs on to boil and had served up the potatoes. Now he was taking the eggs off the stove.

Through supper Jenny sat in her mother's chair with her head down listening to Jimmy tell Evan how, when old man

Hoover's wife scolded him for bringing mud into the kitchen, he had slapped her, knocking her across the room. Jenny was shocked, and thought of her father, who could be pretty cranky. He never hit any of them or her mother.

Now she was reminded of the book and the husband who expected his wife to have everything perfect for him but never thanked her. Indeed he would threaten her with a beating. Jenny was glad their home was not like that. But still she remembered her mother looking guilty when she heard her husband coming and hiding the book she was reading while the dirty dishes still sat on the table. Yet he would sit for hours in his big chair, reading his papers, while she worked in the kitchen.

Jenny thought of Shammy, wondering what he'd be like as a husband. But why think of him? He was more interested in the new teacher. He had passed right by her today without even a smile; he was so busy being a cowboy. How would the teacher like to be a housewife, maybe teaching as well to bring money into the home, as Jenny's mother had done for many years? Ordinarily Jenny never thought much about her mother but everything seemed to be coming to her attention today. She saw her mother's life as hard, with little free time.

"My shoulder is hurting, Evan," she said, wanting to say, "and my period is getting me down" just for fun. Instead saying, "I think I'll go to bed."

YEAST INFECTIONS

Yeast infections are annoying infections that can occur in your vulva and vagina. Unfortunately they are also common. Other names for yeast infections are *candida, monilia* or *yeast fungus.*

You know you have a yeast infection when some or all of these symptoms occur ...

- your crotch is very itchy, red, raw, sore and/or irritated
- it burns slightly when you pee
- your vaginal secretions smell very strongly like baking bread
- your vaginal secretions are white and thick like cottage cheese or yoghurt
- you feel exhausted

Fortunately there's relief. First, go to your doctor to make sure that you have a yeast infection and not something more serious. Then go to the drugstore and get some of the soothing anti-yeast suppositories made just for yeast infections. These are inserted into the vagina and can be messy but they sure make you feel better. Be certain to follow the directions and use *all* the medication to completely clear up the infection.

Yeast infections are caused when there is a change in the *pH chemical balance* of your vagina. This might happen for a number of reasons, such as menstruation, the use of some antibiotics and birth control

(cont'd)

pills, diabetes and pregnancy. In these situations, the yeast — which is always present in your vagina — may grow out of control.

You can protect yourself by drinking a big glass of cranberry juice a day or by eating all natural unsweetened yoghurt. Wear cotton underwear instead of synthetic materials. Be sure to always wipe from the front of your vulva to the back when you're finished going to the bathroom to make sure yeast from your anus (where you have bowel movements) doesn't get into your vagina. If you have a yeast infection, plain yogurt applied to your vagina may soothe the itching although it won't necessarily clear up the infection.

Thirteen and Normal

CARMEN RODRÍGUEZ

TRANSLATED FROM THE SPANISH BY
LORI NORDSTROM WITH CARMEN RODRÍGUEZ

In "Thirteen and Normal," Carmen Rodríguez writes about growing up in Chile in the early 1960s. Cecilia, the hero, is frustrated at what being a girl seems to mean. She doesn't like the awkward equipment that goes with getting her period. She doesn't like her mother's curfews and lectures. And she especially doesn't like having to do housework. In spite of her frustrations, Cecilia finds comfort in an unexpected friend.

Monday, October 7, 1961

I'm thirteen years old and I think I'm normal. I like a boy named Alberto and I think he likes me too. Well, at least that's what my friends Gloria and Doris say. But they probably just say it to make me feel better because, the truth is,

Alberto has never paid any attention to me. He has never spoken to me and every time I see him in the hall or the schoolyard he's fooling around with his friends and doesn't even realize I exist.

My friends say that I'm being stupid, that I have to take more initiative and at least let Alberto know that I like him. But I'm scared stiff. My mom's always going on about how girls must be careful not to become "easy prey" for men. I would never say anything to her about it because she would probably slap me, but when she talks about being "easy prey" for men all I can think of are the birds of prey we learned about in Science. And then I think of myself as a little mouse running through tall grass and Alberto as an eagle, swooping down on me, closer and closer, until he finally sinks his claws into my furry little body. When I think about stuff like that I get a weird feeling. I don't know how to explain it but it's like a burning feeling between my legs; it's like burning and throbbing at the same time and I'm getting kind of sick of feeling it too. I don't know if it's normal. Maybe I'm not normal. I should ask Gloria and Doris about it, but I'm too embarrassed.

Tuesday, October 8, 1961

While I was drying the dishes after dinner tonight, my mom gave me this big long lecture. She said that boys like to take advantage of girls, that they only think about "one thing," and that girls must be very careful not to let boys "get their dirty paws on them." And then I couldn't help but imagine Alberto as a big hairy beast, like a giant gorilla with burning red eyes and huge fangs, standing up on his hind legs and thrashing around his big hairy paws with their long pointy claws. Like King Kong.

And then King Kong Alberto comes crashing through the schoolyard, roaring furiously, and everyone screams and runs for their life, except for me. I am paralysed with terror, motionless. Of course, if we were in the schoolyard, I would look ridiculous because I would be wearing my school uniform and who ever heard of a boy getting his dirty paws on a girl in a uniform? No, not in the schoolyard. On the boulevard that runs along the riverside, instead. On a Sunday.

Now, here comes King Kong Alberto, roaring and foaming at the mouth. Some people scream and run, others dive into the river. The earth trembles, the water grows rough. I am paralysed. I am wearing the pink linen dress my mother sewed for me, my white shoes with a bit of a heel and the matching purse. I am with Gloria and Doris, but they have already jumped into the river, terrified. Oh! I better decide on the underwear I have on because King Kong Alberto is sure to rip my pink dress to shreds. Which is too bad, really, because I do like it a lot. Okay, I'm wearing the bikini panties and lace bra set that I bought with my own money and that my mom says is for whores. I don't have a slip to go with it, so I'll have to wear the white cotton one with the crocheted hem that my grandma gave me. Yes, that's the prettiest one.

And so, I'm paralysed, leaning back against a tree, and I see Alberto King Kong coming closer, staring at me with his huge red eyes and baring his huge pointy fangs. I feel like I'm hypnotized, because I know he's about to scoop me up into his dirty paws....

I was already starting to feel the burning between my legs when my mom started yelling at me because I wasn't paying any attention to her, as usual. She said she's sure ALL other girls wished they had a mother like her, concerned about her daughter and prepared to give her advice. And then she went on and on about how when SHE was a girl, nobody warned her about anything and bla bla bla, and then she started to cry. I guess I sort of felt sorry for her but I was already too mad. She's always yelling at me for nothing and babbling on and on. Besides, she treats me like I'm stupid. So I threw the dish towel on the floor and ran out of the kitchen and up to my room. I even slammed the door behind me.

And here I am now, writing to you, dear diary, because you are the only one who understands me. I don't know what to do, because maybe my mom is right and all that boys want is to take advantage of girls. But then I don't understand anything because where does love fit into all of this? Could it be that men don't feel love? Or maybe the ones who do don't touch the girls they love. But in the movies, whenever a man and a woman fall in love, they always kiss and touch each other. I just don't understand at all. I'll have to talk to Gloria and Doris about this.

◉ Putting It All Together ◉

Thursday, October 10, 1961

Today Gloria brought a book called *The Positions of Love* to school. At recess we locked ourselves into the bathroom to look at it and almost peed ourselves laughing. It's a good thing we were in the bathroom!

I thought that men's things were hairy, but it seems they're not, only their balls are hairy. But the most disgusting thing was when ... oh, dear diary, I can't even say it, but you're the only one I can speak freely with. Okay, the most disgusting thing was when ... she was sucking it! Yuck! I could NEVER have imagined something so disgusting! I'm sure my mom and dad never did anything like that. And I will never do it. Ever. But Gloria says that when you're in love, you will do ANYTHING and that this is the most natural thing in the world. I don't believe it. Besides, it can't be healthy. Imagine all those germs. How disgusting.

After looking at the book I tried to imagine how Alberto would look bare naked. He looks so cute with his clothes on but I've never seen him in a bathing suit. Gloria says that men's things are the same size as their feet, so you should look for a husband with big feet. But I think if it was really big it would hurt.

When I got home I locked myself in the bathroom with my mom's hand mirror, the one she keeps on her dresser. I sat on the toilet and was looking at myself down there, you know where, but I didn't see any hole big enough for a man's thing to fit in. Gloria says there are two holes, one for pee and one for a man's thing to go in and for your period and babies to come out. Just thinking about it makes me hurt, but I also kind of get that burning feeling. I can't be normal.

Today, Miss Blanca told us to read *María* by Jorge Isaacs. She was explaining that it was a novel from Colombia and that it was written during the Romantic Era. Then we started to talk about what "romantic" means, and then we went on to talk about love and stuff like that. Miss Blanca is really cool and in her class you can talk freely about a lot of things because they're part of literature. Gloria said that true love encompasses everything, both spiritual and carnal. Everybody laughed, except for Miss Blanca. When it was my turn to give my opinion, I didn't dare say much, because the truth is, I don't know anything. The only thing I said was that true love was forever. Well, at least that's what the storybooks say. And storybooks must know more than I do.

Saturday, October 12, 1961

So many things have happened, dear diary, that I don't even know where to begin. Well, first of all, Alberto told me that he likes me. Second, I got my period. And third, I had a huge fight with my mom. I want to die. My mom doesn't let me go anywhere and I have to walk around with this big pillow between my legs. My stomach hurts and I haven't seen Alberto for thirty-seven hours and seventeen minutes. I've just been locked up here in my room, crying. My mom brings me food but I don't want to eat. And because she knows that sooner or later I have to leave my room to go to the bathroom and change my pad or go pee, she waits out in the hallway so she can start lecturing me. Stupid old hag! I hate her! Why can't she just leave me alone? Why doesn't she let me live my own life? Just because she's unhappy and my dad left her, she wants me to be the same way she is. That's what I yelled at her yesterday and she started crying, the old cow.

I'm so confused. Everything happened because Alberto walked me to the corner and gave me a kiss. The old cow was watching from the window and she slapped me when I walked into the house. I was still walking on clouds after Alberto's kiss and then smack! I hate her. She doesn't want me to see Alberto, so she hasn't let me go out at all.

And that's not all; it gets worse. Last night I woke up all wet and sticky and I almost died when I saw all that blood! Yes, I got my first period. Thank God I knew about periods because Gloria and Doris already got theirs and had told me about it. I had to get up in the middle of the night and wash myself up. I didn't want to tell my mom but I had to wash the sheets too so she found out anyway. I put a thick pile of folded toilet paper in my panties but today my mom went out and bought sanitary pads. They're like little towels and the most disgusting thing is that you have to wash them after. When my mom left the house I thought of sneaking out but my stomach hurt too much.

Oh, dear diary, what am I going to do? I love him! I love him! And he loves me! After school, I was coming down Pérez Rosales Street when I felt someone's hand on my shoulder. I turned around and ... it was Alberto! I almost died!

He said, "Did you know that I like you a lot?" I felt my face burning, but not nearly as much as the burning and throbbing between my legs. I didn't say anything because I really don't know what you're supposed to say at times like that. Besides, my heart was beating so fast that I was literally choking.

Then he said, "Do you want to go around with me?"

Gloria and Doris had told me that you should always play hard to get and say, "I'll think about it." But I blurted out "Okay" without even realizing it. That was when we got to the corner, and I said, "I live over there." And he said, "Yeah, I know."

And then … he held my chin up and … he kissed me! By that time I was sweating like a pig. I still had my eyes closed when he said, "Are you going to the plaza tonight?"

I said, "Yes."

Him: "At seven?"

Me: "Yes."

Him: "See you there."

Me: "Yes."

Him and me: "Bye."

And then, the stupid old cow said that I wasn't going anywhere all weekend. I hate her. What am I going to do?

Sunday, October 13, 1961

Oh, dear diary, sometimes I think I should leave home, but I don't have anywhere to go. I don't know what to do. Alberto must think I don't like him.

✺ Putting It All Together ✺

Today I finished reading *María* by Jorge Isaacs. I bawled my eyes out. I even got the hiccups. Of course María and Efraín never even kiss, even though they are so in love. Maybe that's what true love is. Maybe my mom is right. Maybe Alberto only wants "that thing." He probably thinks I'm easy and that's why he kissed me right off the bat. But I don't know how you can be in love and not want to kiss the person you love. The book doesn't say anything about whether María wanted to kiss Efraín. I think she did want to and the book just doesn't say anything. I'd like to know what Miss Blanca thinks.

My mom says I'm bleeding a lot for someone so young. I'm probably going to die. Like María. I wish. That would give the old witch something to cry about. And if I died, I wouldn't have to keep thinking about love, or Alberto, or anything. Besides, I'm really fed up with this period stuff. I can't imagine, never mind having to, wash all those stupid pads. Just the thought of it makes me want to die on the spot. Dear diary, if you don't hear from me again, it's because I'm dead.

Monday, October 14, 1961

I didn't die. Today my mom had no choice but to let me go to school. Alberto completely ignored me at recess. I didn't have the nerve to go up to him so I just watched him from a distance. He didn't even do that much. I spent the whole Science period in the bathroom, crying. Then I decided to write him a letter. I had to write about four letters before I got it right. The right one said:

Dear Alberto: (First I had written "My beloved Alberto," but Gloria said it was going too far.) *I did-n't go to the plaza the other day because I was sick all weekend* (which IS true). *If you want, you can walk me to the corner of my house after school.* (I figured we could stop just before we got to the corner so that my mom wouldn't see us.) *Your girlfriend, Cecilia.*

Gloria gave him the letter during the second recess. I didn't go out for recess because I was too embarrassed. After school, I went straight out to the street and waited around awhile before starting to walk home. And you know what, dear diary? Alberto left school with his friends and took off with them in the opposite direction. He didn't even look at me! I couldn't stop crying all the way home and when I got to the corner of my house, my mom was standing right there, the old cow. Which means that if Alberto had walked me home, she would have seen us coming down the street together and she probably would have made a big scene. I barely got in the door when she started lecturing me about how it's not worth it to cry over a boy. I came straight to my room and slammed the door.

I want to die. I haven't stopped bleeding and I can't stand walking around with the bundle between my legs any more. Why did I have to be born a woman? Why??? I want to die. Or maybe I'm not normal and that's why I feel like this.

⊚ Putting It All Together ⊚

Wednesday, October 16, 1961

Alberto is still ignoring me. My period is over. My mom does nothing but cry. I do nothing but cry. Gloria and Doris are being bitches. They start whispering things to each other and then they act all innocent when I come along. Plus, I did really badly on my Science test. The only thing I like is Spanish class because Miss Blanca explains everything really well and she's so nice.

Yesterday I stayed in the classroom during recess because why should I go out if Alberto just ignores me and Gloria and Doris don't want to talk to me? I was the only one in the classroom and I was looking out the window at a piece of sky you can see between the school and the building next door, when I realized that Miss Blanca had walked in. I was crying. She said that if I needed somebody to talk to I could talk to her. I just shook my head. I'm too embarrassed. What am I supposed to say to her? That I don't want to be a girl? That I want to die? She would realize right away that I'm not normal and then she might hold it against me and give me bad marks in Spanish, the only subject I'm doing well in. What am I going to do?

Sunday, October 20, 1961

Another weekend without being allowed to go out alone. At least we went to my grandma's for tea today. Otherwise I would've gone crazy locked up inside all day. Crazier. On top of everything else, my mom made me wash and wax all the floors in the house. Why did I have to be born a girl?

My grandma loves me, I know she loves me. Maybe I could go and live with her. But in spite of everything, I feel sorry for my mom. I couldn't leave her alone. Today my grandma was telling me that all girls should learn how to bake bread and cakes and pies, and that she was going to teach me. The truth is that I couldn't care less. But I had to smile and say yes because the poor old thing would die if I told her to get lost. I'm going to start going there every Saturday afternoon so that she can teach me. At least I can get out of the house and get some fresh air.

My mom is just thrilled about the whole idea. I felt like telling her that if she thinks it's so great maybe she should be the one to learn. In fact, in my whole life, I have never seen her bake anything except those awful cookies that look like shoe soles and taste like medicine. Stupid cow. Why was I born a woman? As if my damned period and my broken heart and waxing all the floors weren't enough, now I have to learn how to bake bread and cakes and pies ....

Oh, dear diary, the truth is that I am totally confused. Why did Alberto stop liking me? I've cried so much that I have no tears left. Or maybe it's just that I don't like Alberto that much any more. It probably wasn't true love. But, when I think about that kiss he gave me, I start to sweat. But that must be because I'm not normal. Good night.

Wednesday, October 23, 1961
You'll never guess what happened! All hell broke loose! Mrs Marta, the Math teacher, caught Gloria and Doris in

the bathroom with that love positions book. It looks like they're going to get expelled. It's a good thing that I'm not friends with them any more although that stupid Gloria almost got me into trouble too. She tried to tell Mrs Marta that I also liked those kind of books or something like that. But, lucky for me, Mrs Marta didn't buy it and told her to keep her mouth shut. Then she gave the class this big lecture while she waved the book around like a flag saying, "These young ladies read por-no-gra-phic literature!" Then she took them off to the principal's office.

We had Spanish next period so we asked Miss Blanca what "pornographic literature" was. She blushed a little bit at first but then she explained that it means obscene literature, books and magazines that use human bodies for bad reasons, usually to make money. I raised my hand and said that maybe the book that Gloria and Doris had was not porno-graphic because it was about love and what two people do when they're in love. The whole class started laughing but Miss Blanca didn't laugh. She winked at me and said that she hadn't seen the book herself so she really couldn't say one way or the other.

After class, when everyone else had already left the room, Miss Blanca came up to me. She asked how I was. I said I was better. She asked if what was bothering me had anything to do with love.

"I don't know," I said. "Maybe. But the worst thing is that I don't want to be a girl. I hate having periods and hav-ing to learn to bake bread and pies and having to wax the floors, just because I'm a girl. And on top of it all, I don't know if boys like me or if they just want to take advantage of me. I can't stand being a girl. I want to die."

I don't know how I could've said all that to her! I just blurted it all out without even thinking about it! Then I asked her, "Do you think I'm normal?"

Oh, dear diary, then the most amazing thing happened! Miss Blanca took my hands in hers, looked at me with tears in her eyes (yes, she was crying!) and said, "I know how you feel. Sometimes I also get tired of being a woman. Sometimes I also feel like dying. But I don't think there's anything wrong with you or me. You and I are the normal ones."

Yes, that's what she said: "You and I are the normal ones." Oh, dear diary, I practically flew home, floating along, light as a feather! I even gave my mom a kiss when I got home. And the best part is, I don't feel like dying any more. I'm normal! I'm normal!

Saturday, October 26, 1961

Today I went to my grandma's to learn how to make bread. I walked there alone, so I got a chance to go by the plaza on the way, but there was nobody there. Grandma had the woodstove going and had made tea. So we had a few cups of tea while we were making the bread. I love Grandma's kitchen because it's really big and it's always nice and warm. She has all these dried herbs and things hanging all over and a big huge table where she does everything.

◉ Putting It All Together ◉

Baking bread is pretty easy but you have to learn how to give it "the right touch" so that it doesn't come out too soft in the middle and too crusty on the outside. The best part is kneading. Kneading and kneading the dough, which is soft and tough at the same time, pushing down on it with the palm of your hands, squeezing it between your fingers, stretching it out and kneading it all over again.

When I was kneading the dough, I started to feel that burning feeling between my legs again, and then because the oven was on and the kitchen was so warm, I started sweating like a pig. Grandma looked over at me and she asked me if I was feeling all right and why was I so flushed. I told her I was just hot. What else could I say? Maybe I'm not normal after all.

Sunday, October 27, 1961

Today my mom let me go to the plaza. I hung around with Rina Ramírez. Gloria and Doris are grounded because they almost got expelled. I was walking around with Rina when this boy from grade ten came up to me. I think his name is Manuel. He's really cute, black hair, green eyes. That stupid Rina nudged me with her elbow so hard I'm sure the whole world saw. Then she got the giggles. I almost got the giggles too but I managed to control myself.

Anyway, Manuel invited me to the school's basketball game next Wednesday. He plays left forward on the school team. My mom has never let me go to a game so I've never seen him play, but Rina says he's really good. I told him I would go, but I don't know what I'm going to do. My mom will never let me go. Maybe I can tell her that I'm going to Rina's to study Math. Oh diary, what am I going to do?

CYSTITIS

Bladder infections are diseases related to urinating (going pee). The bladder is the organ in which urine is stored. The most common bladder infection is *cystitis.*

You know you have cystitis when you have to urinate every few minutes but very little pee comes out. When it does come out, it often feels like you're burning to death! You may also find blood on the toilet paper when you wipe. Some women smell a strong odour in their urine and find that their urine is cloudy.

If you notice the infection early enough and if you're in good health, you can treat it yourself by drinking lots and lots of liquid, especially water and unsweetened cranberry juice, but *don't* drink beverages with caffeine or alcohol! When you pee, empty your bladder completely and always go to the bathroom when you have the urge.

(cont'd)

However, if you find you're in a lot of pain or can't clear up your infection, go to the doctor or hospital emergency room as soon as possible. It is very important to get rid of bladder infections because they can lead to further infections that are life-threatening. The doctor will give you antibiotics that will clear up the symptoms quickly. Be sure to take *all* of the presribed medication

There are lots of ways to protect yourself from bladder infections. If you wear pads when you menstruate, wash often because the bloody pad can carry infection causing bacteria from your anus (where you have bowel movements) to travel to your vagina, causing yeast infections, or to your urethra (where you urinate) causing bladder infections. (See diagram page 28.) When you're going to the bathroom, always wipe from front to back. If you're sexually active, make sure you're well lubricated before having sex and try to urinate immediately after sex, because this flushes out the urethra.

Character Building

EMMY PANTIN

Emmy Pantin is a high school student. In "Character Building," Emmy sifts through advice from her mother, conversations with friends, and her own insights. She is trying to understand the relationship between menstruating and growing up a woman. Emmy neither glorifies her periods nor is disgusted by them, but comes to respect and appreciate the strength and power of her body.

WHAT DEFINES ME IS THE strength of my character. This is what my mother taught me about menstruating. Others have said that their mothers told them menstruation would hurt, that it would go on forever, that they would need special products to cope, that they were doomed to a life forever struggling with The Curse. Some mothers told their daughters nothing at all — one of my friends thought she was bleeding to death until the school nurse explained things to her. But like fathers telling their sons about competing in sports or building things with tools, my mother told me that bleeding would "build character."

I have never hated my period, even after my male cousin shrieked, "What's that smell?" when I had just discarded a blood-soaked pad in the bathroom. His disgust at the whole idea of menstruation only made me more proud. I never wanted to be one of the boys.

My mother wanted to throw a party when, at thirteen, I told her that I had finally gotten IT. She hugged me and, predictably, told me that I was a big girl and would be all grown up before I knew it. I didn't undergo the extreme metamorphoses I had been led to believe would occur. I expected a new appreciation for high heels and children. Instead, I continued to play schoolyard games on concrete playgrounds, patiently waiting for the day I would Grow Up.

Lately I've found myself in estrogen-based bonding sessions with friends. They recite long lists of complaints against their bodies. Menstruation is discussed and vehemently cursed for all its evil symptoms: cramps, bloodstains, bloating, pimples, weight gain, backaches, increased sex drive (or the opposite), tenderness, sensitivity, mood swings, PMS. I feel entirely left out and I wonder if this means I haven't yet grown up.

While I have experienced some of these symptoms I've never referred to myself as someone who "suffers" because of them. Sometimes friends react to my alienation on the subject of menstrual pain with: "You're not a woman then!" But I am a woman and I bleed like the rest of them.

I've talked to my mother about the hatred my friends seem to feel towards their bodies and specifically the female functions, and she nods her head in agreement. "I know. A lot of women complain about their bodies. What they don't know is that their periods are what gives them strength, what makes them powerful. Women have been taught to hate their bodies and to see their periods as a curse. It's not a curse. It's a gift."

I believe other women when they say they're in pain. Yet I can't help but feel as though some of my friends show a real disrespect to their bodies when they say they'd give up their period if they had the choice. If I had the choice, my menstruating is the last thing I'd give up. My mother taught me that just because you bleed once a month doesn't mean you're weak or any less than a man. In fact, she told me, it means that you're stronger if you carry on despite any pain. That's the esteem in which I was taught to hold menstruation, and that's the way I will always look at it. It doesn't make me any less than a man — it makes me more.

I look down the road and realize that I won't have my period forever. What will it mean when I stop menstruating? Will it mean I am no longer a woman? Will I become asexual? Will I be like a man?

My mother started menopause in her late forties just when I was starting my period. I asked her what it all meant and she told me, "Menopause is when you stop having your period. It means you can't have babies any more."

"Is having babies what makes me a woman?"

◎ Putting It All Together ◎

My mother thought about this for a moment and replied, "You aren't defined by the babies you have. You're defined by your own strength. When your period stops, you'll be even wiser because you'll have gone through an experience that others haven't gone through. Menopause isn't the end of something, it's the beginning of something else. Few roles are defined for older women the way they are for younger women, so the end of your period is kind of like the beginning of a new life that hasn't yet been defined."

During dinner with four friends yesterday we discovered that we were all on our periods at that same time. I wonder how that happens. Maybe because we've been together for so long our minds and bodies have begun to function on the same cycle. We can finish each other's sentences, we can guess with incredible accuracy each other's behavior in any given situation, and now we menstruate at the same time. We have grown into a rhythm together and I wonder if, although none of us wears high heels or yearns for children, maybe this is what becoming a woman really means. We are growing up together, having dinner in a restaurant, discovering that we are linked through the blood that flows from our bodies.

I'm nineteen now and that magical transformation that was supposed to suddenly occur once I got my period hasn't come yet. As a woman I don't want to fit into any moulds that are set out for me by anyone other than myself. I align myself with other women, but I define myself through my own insight. In the meantime, I carry on with my life and continue to build character, add strength and knowledge to the person I am becoming. I like what I've got so far, menstrual cramps and all.

Period Days

Mark your bleeding days on this calendar. Use your favourite coloured marker!
After a while, you may notice a pattern to your monthly cycles.

Length of cycle		1	2	3	4	5	6	7	8	9	10	11	12	13	14	15	16	17	18	19	20	21	22	23	24	25	26	27	28	29	30	31
	JANUARY																															
	FEBRUARY																															
	MARCH																															
	APRIL																															
	MAY																															
	JUNE																															
	JULY																															
	AUGUST																															
	SEPTEMBER																															
	OCTOBER																															
	NOVEMBER																															
	DECEMBER																															

Do you experience certain sensations before or during your period? Mark on the calendar the days that you experience period signs like mood swings, cramps or vivid dreams. Use special symbols or letters for each sensation: C = cramps or * = dreams

At the end of each month, think about your eating habits, how much you exercised and how stressful your life has been. Is there a connection between your bleeding patterns and your life style?

Other Books You Might Want Read About This Crazy Time In Your Life

Finding Our Way: The Teen Girls' Survival Guide — Allison Abner and Linda Villarosa, with Queen Latifah; New York: Harper Perennial, 1995.

Changing Bodies, Changing Lives — Ruth Bell and other editors; New York: Random House, 1980, 1987.

Are You There God? It's Me, Margaret — Judy Blume; Scarsdale, New York: Bradbury Press, 1970.

How Sex Works — Elizabeth Fenwick and Richard Walker; London; New York: Dorling Kindersley, 1994.

Period — JoAnn Gardner-Loulan, Bonnie Lopez and Marcia Quackenbush; San Francisco: Volcano Press, 1981.

The Period Book — Karen Gravelle and Jennifer Gravelle; New York: Walker & Co., 1996.

It's Perfectly Normal! — Robie Harris; Cambridge, Massachusetts: Candlewick Press, 1994.

What's Happening to My Body for Girls — Lynda Madaras; New York: Newmarket Press, 1987.

Bringing Up Parents: The Teenager's Handbook — Alex J. Packer; Minneapolis, Minnesota: Free Spirit Publications, 1992.

It's OK to Be You — Claire Patterson and Lindsay Quilter; Berkeley, California: Tricycle Press, 1994.

GLOSSARY

A NOTE ON SLANG TERMS: Some of the definitions in this glossary include slang words. Sometimes people are so shy of their bodies and of sex that they make up silly words, or other times they just don't know what the correct words are. People also use slang when they think the correct words sound boring or too medical. This sure can create a lot of confusion! There are many, many slang words for our bodies and sex so we've only been able to include a few. Slang is often disrespectful and offensive so we highly recommend using the real words when you talk about your body.

AMENORRHEA: The medical term that is used when a woman or a girl's periods stop altogether. Amenorrhea may be caused by a number of things: too much dieting, poor eating habits, illness, being on the birth control pill, pregnancy or menopause.

ANEMIA: People with anemia feel weak and tired all of the time and have problems with concentration. Anemia occurs when there is not enough of the mineral iron in your body. Heavy menstrual periods or poor eating habits can make you anemic.

ANOREXIA (ANOREXIA NERVOSA): A very dangerous medical condition that occurs when a person diets so much that she's no longer healthy. People with anorexia are very afraid of getting fat and, while often very, very thin, see themselves as overweight. Anorexic women and girls often stop having their menstrual periods. Anorexia is life-threatening.

ANUS: It's from this opening that you have bowel movements (poo). The anus is between the buttocks of both men and women. Slang: butthole, bum.

BLOATING: A condition that makes areas of the body swell. Bloating is caused by water retention. Before your period, hormonal changes may cause your body to hold back some of the water that you would usually pee or sweat out. Your belly, breasts, even your fingers can bloat.

CERVIX: The narrow opening that acts as the gateway between the vagina and the uterus. When a pregnant woman gives birth, the cervix must dilate, or open up, so that the baby can come out.

CLITORIS: This tiny, bud-shaped organ is located outside of a woman's body at the top of her labia. It's protected by folds of skin and when touched in certain ways will feel pleasurable. See also: Masturbation. Slang: clit, button.

CRAMPS: Pains in the lower abdomen (just below your tummy) that can occur during or before menstruation. No one knows for certain why this happens, but doctors think that it may be linked to poor eating habits (too much fatty food and not enough fibre and vegetables in our diets) and too little exercise. See also: Dysmenorrhea.

CYCLE (MENSTRUAL CYCLE): A cycle is a process that repeats itself over and over again. The menstrual cycle is made up of a number of different stages, all of which are directed by the body's hormones. The length of a menstrual cycle varies from woman to woman and can be from twenty to forty days long. The average cycle is twenty-eight days.

DISCHARGE (SECRETIONS): The sticky white or clear mucus that you may find on your underwear. Each day it's produced by your cervix and vagina to wash your internal organs, keeping them clean and free of infection. A woman's vagina also produces discharge when she gets sexually excited. This discharge acts as a lubricant during sex.

DYSMENORRHEA: The medical term for Cramps.

EGG (OVUM): The female reproductive cell. The ovaries contain tiny eggs (ova). Once menstruation begins, an egg is released from one of the ovaries each cycle. Pregnancy occurs when an egg meets up with a sperm after sexual intercourse.

EJACULATION: The release of sperm from a man's penis. Slang: to come, coming.

EMBRYO: The medical term for the developing cells during the first eight weeks of pregnancy. If the pregnancy continues, these cells will later become a baby.

ENDOMETRIUM: The blood and mucus lining that grows in the uterus during the first stage of the menstrual cycle. Menstrual "blood" is a mixture of mucus and secretions from the vagina and the cervix with the blood and mucus of the endometrium.

ERECTION: When a boy or a man has an erection, his penis expands in size and becomes hard so that it sticks out from his body. This usually happens when he is sexually excited. But boys who are going through puberty can have erections even when they are not sexually excited. An erection can last for a few minutes or up to an hour. Slang: boner, hard-on.

FALLOPIAN TUBE: The passageway between each ovary and the uterus. Following ovulation, the egg leaves the ovary and travels down the fallopian tube into the uterus.

GENITALS: This word is used in a general way to describe the sexual and reproductive organs that are on the outside of a person's body. This word is used for both men and women. A woman's genitals include her clitoris, labia and the opening of her vagina. (See also Vulva.) A man's genitals include his scrotum and penis. Slang: private parts, down there, crotch.

HIV/AIDS: AIDS is a life-threatening disease that affects people's immune system, making them vulnerable to certain illnesses. AIDS is believed to be caused by the HIV virus, which is transmitted through the bodily fluids: semen, blood, including menstrual blood, vaginal discharge or breast milk. People can protect themselves from HIV/AIDS by using condoms when they have oral sex or penetrative sex. You cannot get HIV/AIDS from kissing or hugging.

HORMONES: Hormones are messages that your body and brain send back and forth so that each part of your body knows what to do. Hormones are always flowing through your body, but there are many more of them during puberty when your body is maturing and learning new processes and sensations. Estrogen and progesterone are the female sex hormones.

HYMEN: The thin membrane that protects the vagina when a girl is quite young. Most girls' hymens are usually separated or "torn" during sports or by using tampons, while others' hymens are stretched during heavy petting or sexual intercourse.

LABIA: The folds of skin that protect the vagina (the fleshy skin between your legs). As you physically mature, the labia become softer and looser. Slang: lips.

MASTURBATION: The term used when people give themselves sexual pleasure by touching their genitals. A girl or a woman masturbates by touching her clitoris, vagina and breasts. A boy or a man touches his penis and testicles. Masturbation is normal and most people do it even though the topic is often considered embarrassing or bad in our society. Slang: (for a woman) playing with yourself, getting off; (for a man) beating off, jacking off.

MENARCHE: Pronounced "men-ark-ie," this is the medical term for first menstruation.

MENOPAUSE: The end of menstruation, which generally occurs when a women is in her early fifties. Women can no longer become pregnant once they reach menopause. Slang: the change.

MENSES: Another word for menstruation.

MENSTRUATION: For a few days each month a woman or a girl will bleed from her vagina. This bleeding time is called menstruation and can last two to seven days. Menstruation will happen when a girl begins to mature into adulthood, anywhere from age nine to sixteen. Once a girl begins menstruating, the bleeding will usually return every twenty to forty days. Slang: period, visitor, friend, that time of the month, the curse.

OVARIES: The thumbnail-sized organs that produce eggs (ova). There are two ovaries, one on the left and one on the right side of the uterus. Once a month one ovary releases an egg that travels through the fallopian tube to the uterus.

OVULATION: The medical term for the time during each menstrual cycle when an ovary releases an egg (ovum). Ovulation usually occurs about fourteen days before your menstrual period.

OVUM: See Egg.

◎ Glossary ◎

PAP SMEAR/TEST: During an annual checkup by a doctor, a sample or "smear" of the secretions and cells of the vagina and cervix are tested for disease or abnormalities.

PERIOD: The common term for menstruation.

PRE-MENSTRUAL SYNDROME: PMS is a term used to describe the sensations a woman may get before her menstruation begins: cramps, backache, headache, increased emotions (anger, sadness, happiness).

PUBERTY: This is the crazy time in a person's life when she (or he) rapidly changes from a child into an adult. Puberty happens to everyone sooner or later. In girls, puberty can begin as early as eight or nine, while in boys, puberty doesn't usually begin until age eleven or twelve. For a young woman, puberty will mean she will get her menstrual period, grow breasts and her hips will widen. For a young man, puberty will cause his voice to deepen, hair to grow on his face and his penis will grow too. Both girls and boys grow taller, grow hair in their armpits and around their genitals, may develop pimples, and will have new feelings about sex. It usually takes about three or four years for these changes to occur. Because it's a time of great physical change, puberty can be kind of confusing emotionally!

SEMEN: The liquid (made up of millions of sperm) that comes out of a man's penis during ejaculation.

SEX/SEXUAL INTERCOURSE: When two people choose to give each other pleasure by touching, kissing and rubbing one another's bodies, particularly the genitals. Sexual inter-course occurs when a man's penis is inserted into a woman's vagina, while penetrative sex can include anal as well as vaginal sex. When a person kisses or licks another person's gentials it's called oral sex. Any sexual activity that is forced on someone against her (or his) will is considered sexual assault and is against the law. Slang: making love, having sex, doing it. Slang for oral sex: blow job, going down.

SPERM: The male reproductive cell. Both the egg and the sperm are needed to create a baby.

TOXIC SHOCK SYNDROME: A rare but life-threatening illness that has been linked to using tampons. Most often women get TSS by wearing tampons too long (they must be changed every four to five hours) or from using tampons that are too absorbent.

URETHRA: It's from this opening that you urinate (pee). In women, the urethra is located between your labia, just ahead of your vaginal opening. In men, the urethra open-ing is at the end of the penis.

UTERUS (WOMB): The uterus is a very strong and muscular hollow organ about the size of your fist. It's located inside your body, just below your belly button. This is where menstrual blood comes from, and it's also the place where a baby grows when a woman is pregnant.

⊚ Glossary ⊚

VAGINA: The spongy tunnel that connects the uterus and cervix with the outside of your body. Your vaginal opening is between the folds of your labia.

VULVA: The word for the area between your legs. Your vulva is made up of your external sex organs, the labia and clitoris, and the vaginal opening. Your pubic hair covers and protects this area.

ABOUT THE AUTHORS

IDA FISHER taught school and counselled for thirty-one years. She is presently auditing courses in the Religion and Culture Department at Wilfrid Laurier University. Although she is legally blind, she leads an active life and enjoys swimming, listening to music and travelling.

JANE EATON HAMILTON is the author of the children's book, *Jessica's Elevator*, two poetry books, *Body Rain* and *Steam-Cleaning Love*, and a collection of short fiction, *July Nights*. *Body Rain* was short-listed for the Pat Lowther Award. *July Nights* was short-listed for the VanCity Award and the Ethel Wilson Fiction Award in the BC Book Prizes.

Since completing her final exams in English Language and Literature at St Edmund Hall, Oxford, COLETTE HARRIS has worked for a small publishing company, taken a post-graduate diploma in journalism, and worked as a freelance journalist for a variety of magazines. She hopes that she is on the way to making a career out of writing.

❁ About the Authors ❁

Raised in Malaysia, MANJIT KAUR finds many of her stories are set there. She is currently an editorial assistant for the literary journal *Prairie Schooner* and is completing an MA in English at the University of Nebraska-Lincoln. Besides writing fiction, she also writes essays and has presented papers at numerous conferences. She hopes to write a novel soon.

LILIAN NATTEL is a Toronto writer whose short stories and poetry have appeared in *Event, Fireweed, Lilith, Parchment, Bridges* and *The Fiddlehead*. She teaches creative writing to senior citizens, who are an inspiration to her. "New Moon" is adapted from "The River Midnight," an adult novel currently in progress about a fictional Polish village.

CHI NGUYEN is a sixteen year old young woman who plans on a career in journalism. She is on the editorial board of *Venus: A Young Women's Health Newsletter* which is published in Toronto. Her sister, Diane, helps type Chi's articles and stories.

KATHLEEN O'GRADY is currently completing her PhD in the area of contemporary Continental philosophy at the University of Cambridge, UK. She has published several journal and book articles in the area of philosophy, religious studies and feminist theory. Her co-edited volume *Bodies, Lives, Voices: Essays in Gender and Theology* is forthcoming (1997) with Sheffield Academic Press.

SUE OSWALD taught English and was coordinator of the professional writing programme at the University of Maryland.

She was born with "multiple congenital defects" which required various treatments and hospitalizations over the years. In 1972, at the age of eleven, she was treated for severe scoliosis. Sue Oswald died in 1997 as a result of complications from surgery and heart failure.

EMMY PANTIN is a high school student who loves to write poetry. She spends much of her time educating her peers on issues like homophobia, racism, HIV/AIDS and STDs.

CARMEN RODRÍGUEZ was born in Chile in 1948 and came to Canada as a political exile in 1974. She is the author of a collection of poetry, *Guerra Prolongada/ Protracted War* (1992), and a collection of short stories, *and a body to remember with* (1997).

Living and working in Edmonton, Alberta, GERMAINE ST. PAUL raised four children as a single parent. Two of her stories were performed and then published in the chapbook *Womanstrength* (1992). Her story "Love Knot" was the frontispiece for the 1993 Alberta Medical Association report on doctor abuse of patients.

KARYN SILZER is a student in her last year of high school. She enjoys playing sports, especially volleyball and basketball, and is very involved in the life of her school through clubs and student council. Her goal is to pursue a career in the field of health studies education.

◎ About the Authors ◎

LOUISE SIMON spent her first fifteen years on a ranch in Alberta; it was there in the late 1920s that she had her first period. She worked as a nursing sister in the RCAF for five years. In 1977, she earned a BA from Bishops University. She began writing poetry and short stories in 1980, and has had her work published in a number of magazines including *Quarry, Room of One's Own* and *Grain,* as well as in the anthology *Celebrating Canadian Women.*

STEPHANIE STEARN is a painter, gardener and hausfrau. Born in England, raised in Toronto, she now lives in Alliston, Ontario.

MARY HELEN STEFANIAK has taught literature and writing in a variety of settings, including an all-girls' high school in Milwaukee, the University of Nebraska in Omaha, and the University of Iowa, where she also worked as fiction editor of *The Iowa Review.* She is the mother of two teenage daughters and one son. Her first book, *Self Storage and Other Stories,* was published in 1997.

TAMARA STEINBORN is a graduate student in English at the University of Manitoba. She has had poetry and critical writing published in *Prairie Fire* and *Room of One's Own.*

ARDELLE STEUERNOL loves to tell stories and those around her enjoy them all: a quiet bedtime story to her grandsons or a full blown tale on a topic past, present or future. She is a two-time winner of the Dorothy Shoemaker literary award and has published in *Voice from the Yellow House.*

ROSEMARY VOGT (née Suderman) was raised on a dairy farm near Niverville, Manitoba in a family of Russian Mennonite background. She lives with her husband, their three children, a dog and a cat, near Steinbach. Presently she is completing a Bachelor's Degree in Education at the University of Winnipeg. In her spare time she writes, travels and enjoys going to live theatre.

PAULA WANSBROUGH is a youth and community worker in downtown Toronto. She teaches sex education, computer and Internet skills and is the former supervising editor of *Venus: A Young Women's Health Newsletter*. She has her MA in Religion and Cultural Studies from Wilfrid Laurier University.

MARY ALICE WARD was born the daughter of an Armenian mother who weaned her on the stories of the Armenian genocide of 1915, and of an Idaho cowboy who made sure she knew how to ride a horse downhill in the desert. She is currently working towards her Master's degree in Religious Studies at the University of Colorado and is a new mother.

ABOUT THE OTHER CONTRIBUTORS

ESMERALDA CARVALHO is a community health educator who presents sexuality and AIDS workshops.

DIANE DRIEDGER is a poet, writer, historian and disability activist. Her most recent book is *Across Borders: Women with Disabilities Working Together* (1996).

BRANDY FORD is twenty-two. She has had several poems and short stories published and has written regularly for the local newspaper. Presently she lives in Welland, Ontario and is writing a children's book.

ATHENA GEORGE lives on Salt Spring Island, British Columbia. She attended the writing programme at David Thompson University Centre in Nelson, British Columbia. In 1984, the provincial government closed this arts university.

RUTH HELLIWELL is a happily married retired nurse who keeps busy by grandmothering ten beautiful grandchildren, doing volunteer work and travelling.

ROBERTA KENNEDY is a Haida and Squamish woman originally from Haida Gwaii (aka Queen Charlotte Islands). She is a university graduate who now lives in Victoria, British Columbia.

Ninety-three year old URSULA KROFT remembers when she climbed trees and chased balls. Her aunt would scold her saying such behaviour was not fit for a girl, but Ursula used to retort (and still says) "I like fun too!"

Seventeen year old CLAUDIA MARQUES will soon graduate from high school. She loves working as a tutor for newly immigrated high school students because she vividly remembers the trials she faced when her family moved to Canada from Portugal.

YOLANDE BÉLANGER MENNIE is a freelance writer and editor. She earns her keep by writing and editing for international development organizations and women's groups. She also writes articles, stories and poems for the pleasure of it.

ELIZABETH MOSSMAN is a visual artist who paints with acrylic and oil, does quilt-making and printmaking, and lives in Boulder, Colorado.

TIFFANIE NEILSON is sixteen years old and a peer sexuality educator in schools and community centres. She lives with her mother and two insane cats.

RUBINA RAMJI is a PhD student in Religious Studies. She was born in East Africa but has lived most of her life in Canada.

◎ About the Other Contributors ◎

CAROLYN SAUNDERS lives in Vancouver, British Columbia and is proud to say she knows nothing about skiing, golfing or boating.

DR DEBRA WIENS lives with her husband and two daughters. She practises family medicine with an interest in psychiatry. Her personal interests include music, mythology and the theatre.

RUTH WOOD is a photo-carrying granny who lives in Winnipeg, Manitoba, enjoys quilting and reading CanLit, and supports herself by nursing.

SUSAN, JANTI, JEANANNE and MAJA are in grade eight. They shared their views on menstruation with Paula Wansbrough in a fast-paced and rowdy session.

INDEX

ABOUT KATHLEEN AND PAULA

KATHLEEN O'GRADY is completing her PhD at Trinity College, the University of Cambridge in England. She teaches University courses part-time to help pay for her growing collection of antique marbles. When she isn't writing, reading or teaching, Kathleen spends her days playing with marbles, hoping she hasn't lost any along the way.

PAULA WANSBROUGH is a youth and community worker in downtown Toronto. She teaches sex education, computer and Internet skills and is a former supervising editor of *Venus: A Young Women's Health Newsletter*. She has her MA in Religious Studies from Wilfrid Laurier University. Paula is constantly in awe of the humming complexity of our bodies.